OUR PATH

OUR PATH

A Guide to Navigating the Human Experience

Natasha Tomè

Natasha Tomè

CONTENTS

Do you ever wonder what's the point of it all? The daily routine, the struggle, the mundane parts of your life that feel soul crushing, the disappointment from relationships and family dynamics. Wondering, what did I do to deserve this? Why am I here? Is there more to this life than this? How come others have 'x' and I don't?

If you've ever asked yourself any of these questions, then you've been guided to have this book in your hands at this present moment. Guided by whom you may ask? You'll have that answer by the time you finish reading. There is nothing random about why you're here on Earth at this exact moment in this particular lifetime. And you're not in it alone, the amount of help you have to aid you during this time is astounding. Something we all forget about as soon as we're born.

The problem is, it's not easy being human. With all the different circumstances, families, cultures, friends, and societal dynamics we're exposed to from birth, there's a lot of external stimuli that we have to deal with in addition to trying to figure out who we are, what we want, and what path we can choose for our OWN fulfillment and happiness. While dealing with our fluctuating emotions, thought processes and physical selves. It can be a lot.

But! Life doesn't have to be a constant struggle or just surviving day to day. The Universe would love to see everyone living in a state of self-love, love and compassion for others, abundance, joy and purpose. We can achieve this!

You're about to understand the path of your Soul to help you navigate this lifetime you signed up for.

Let me share with you how this helped my life. I'm second generation Canadian, meaning both my parents immigrated to Canada from Europe with the hope of a better life and more opportunities. So, there was a lot of expectation placed on me, an only child, to follow a prescribed path of success according to family expectations. My parents, God bless them, are hard workers and did their absolute best as they knew how to do. As an adult now, I can see the dysfunctional aspects; the lack of communication, the projection of insecurities, emotional immaturity, and ancestral and familial belief systems I unintentionally absorbed. Compared to some other family units, it really wasn't bad at all, and I am not blaming or complaining. My point is, this meant I grew up with insecurities, low body image, lack of self-love, a lot of self-doubt, a wounded ego, and I allowed my voice to be silenced and became a people pleaser, looking for external validation to boost my self-worth. Not something you consciously realize until you grow up and and start to see the imbalances in your life.

I followed the established route..go to school, attend University, get a stable and safe corporate job, get married, have children and repeat. And this is a path many take happily. It just wasn't for me. After a while, that marriage ended, we didn't have children, the corporate job while abundant, became soul numbing. I got to the point where I was going through the motions, existing, surviving, meeting all my responsibilities and obligations but not finding any real joy or fulfillment in life. The marriage was the first thing to falter, and as some of you may know, divorce is not easy, even if it is amicable. We were going through it and it was a very emotional and stressful time for me, when one day I got a 'random' email about an Angel meditation a local lady was hosting. I say random but really this is one way our helpers communicate with us. So, I went that evening for a meditation outside where a group of us lay on her lawn on yoga mats while she guided us through an Angel meditation, bringing in their energy and healing. Well, I drove home from that meditation feeling the most centred and at peace since we separated. Calm and confident, and sure that this was the best and right path for both of us. I was amazed and thought to myself, I need to find out more about these Angels, this energy we tapped into, from this lady. Thus started an incredible journey into the Spiritual realm and re-awakening of gifts I didn't know I had.

Where was I, up to that point? I had attended a Qigong workshop years earlier and received my first two levels of Reiki certification but didn't practice either outside of the workshop days. I was still very much into a party lifestyle on weekends and my corporate job during the week. That Angel meditation was a real turning point for me, which years later re-awakened psychic abilities and helped me understand just how much help is available to us.

As a result, after much training, study and practice, I left the corporate world and followed my Spiritual path full time. Life has changed dramatically for me, for the better. I am doing work I love, ending ancestral patterns, resolving family issues, and I stopped seeking external validation and feel more fulfilled, happier and at peace within. I am less triggered by the people and circumstances around me and stand in my full power. It's a wonderful feeling. But I'm not going to sugarcoat it, it wasn't an overnight transformation. It took a lot of hard work, self-exploration, tears, angst, backward and forward steps to get here. There were moments that I felt I wasn't improving at all and got tempted to pack it all in and go back to what I knew well and was comfortable with. (That was usually when one of my Spiritual team would give me a big physical sign of encouragement.) I still strive to do better each day, for this human life is a process until we transition back to the Spirit realm. My focus now is to stop my reincarnation cycle and overcome all my Soul challenges and lessons, and at the same time, help others do the same so they can achieve the same kind of freedom. We are Spiritual Beings having a human experience.

And that's the main reason I wrote this book. It's for the novice learning about their real Soul path.

This is a compilation of learning that I've gathered and studied over the years as well as channeled information from various spiritual Beings. My guidance and intent in putting this information together in one book is a taster, a beginner's guide into the world beyond our physical senses, the world that we all come from and will return to. My hope is that you will feel less alone and more optimistic after reading this book and start to realize your own natural power, wisdom and abilities.

I continue to expand my learning by reading, listening, watching, channeling, communicating, and attending events for my own interest and to keep me fresh in all that the Universe provides. I don't claim to know it all but the content contained here is what we need to know now, in order to live our best lives during this human incarnation.

These tips and tools are in addition to the traditional and mainstream resources we have at our disposal; medical doctors, medicine, psychiatrists, psychologists, CBT, counseling, and the multitude of other professionals available to us. What I'm writing about brings us back to the Holistic side, to the army of help we also have available beyond the 3D world.

Really, this book is about Energy. It always comes down to Energy. I touch on each topic to discuss it as simply as possible but each can be further explored by yourself. We cover a huge array of topics and each chapter could be taught as a workshop alone. I'll be offering workshops in the future to go a little deeper into various subjects. If you'd like to be kept informed of those events, please sign up for my newsletter or follow me on social media to stay informed.

In Part One, I explain the background of who we are, where we come from, and the Universe around us. In Part Two, I delve into who are the Beings who can help us, how we can best work with the energy, and practical tips and tools to do so. By the end, I hope you'll have the confidence and knowledge to co-create a fabulous life that is right for you!

Love & Light, Natasha

PART ONE

The Holistic Human and The Universe

1

The Spiritual Soul Path

Energy

We, and the world around us, are nothing but energy and vibrations. Everything in our Universe is energy, vibrating at different levels making things tangible or intangible. It's a Universal Life Force Energy that flows through all living things.

For us humans, if we were to look beyond the superficial layers, beyond the tangible, we'd see each human as a light being, a mass of light full of energy and vibrations. All our light masses are connected by threads of light to one another. Not just to family and loved ones, but to each human on the planet. This contributes to collective consciousness, which we'll explore a little later.
Still looking beyond the surface, we'd also see the trees, rocks, plants, our cars, our homes, and objects represented by vibrating energy at different frequencies to us.

Everything we can see and touch are at their core, energy vibrating at different densities. Not only is the physical represented this way, but also the thoughts, emotions, and words we express. These too have their own energy resonance and make up part of our auric field, which is the energy field we have surrounding our physical bodies. It has also been called our bio plasma or bio field.

Quantum physics has acknowledged that we're all made up of energy, as is everything around us and there are many quotes from renowned physicists and inventors floating around the internet such as; *"we know that everything in life is a vibration"* and *"if you want to find the secrets of the universe, think in terms of energy, frequency and vibration"*, meaning, if you reduce everything down to a subatomic level, everything that exists is based on vibrational frequencies.

We are all individual eternal vibrational vortexes in the Universe and life is a stream of energy in various vibrations, constantly changing, creating and evolving.

Once you understand how much we are, and the world around us, is made up of energy, then you can learn how to be aware of it, work with it, harness it, release it, clear it and co-create a life of fulfillment, abundance, happiness and peace, and a lot more self-love. THAT is the number one priority above all else. Self-love. With the confidence that comes inherent with self-love you will be able to achieve far more than you ever dreamed of.

We are all fields of energetic awareness, we are fully holistic beings, and any imbalance within us affects us on all our levels.

The Google dictionary defines **Holistic** as: *characterized by the belief that the parts of something are interconnected and can be explained only by reference to the whole.*
In terms of healthcare: characterized by the treatment of the whole person, taking into account mental and social factors, rather than just the symptoms of an illness.

The physical, emotional, mental and Spiritual are all aspects of our complete well-being. By the Holistic model, any symptom we have should be examined in all of these areas to determine the root cause and then treat that. Being completely balanced in this way enables us to live an easier life. Let's delve deeper into what a human being consists of.

The Soul

Our Souls are Spirits. We are all Spirits incarnated into a physical shell. At the core of us, we have a Soul. It's an energy light mass that came from a different dimension. Our true inner light is our Soul self. The Soul is an energy and a consciousness, a part of the Divine. Within it, is a Divine spark, an active piece that has come from God, or if you prefer, from Source. Our Souls come from this energy. The physical shell of the human body is just that, a shell, your inner self vibrates with Divine energy, Higher Self consciousness, and light. Your Soul knows your true path and purpose and is never judgmental or critical. It's the part of you that's always connected, always loved. You are never really alone. At least not energetically or Spiritually.

The Divine Spark in the Soul

The Divine spark within your Soul is also called the I AM Presence, that higher aspect, that piece of God within you. It's how you're connected to God and to one another, everyone has a Divine spark within them. When we disconnect from this powerful inner energy, our true self, we feel limitation, lack and worry. You might ask, how do we stay continuously plugged into this energy then? And that there, is the reason for this book. We have so many distractions, obstacles, man made problems, and we're born with the Veil of Amnesia to top it all off!

We share that same Divine spark with every stone, tree, flower, insect, animal, body of water, all of nature, as well as each human, we're all connected on that energetic level.
When we harm nature, an animal, or another human being, we are equally harming ourselves in the same way. This is why there is an epidemic of lack of self-love and self-worth within many humans. Lack of respect for our surroundings and others is a lack of respect for ourselves.

When you make a declaration about yourself, "I AM hungry, tired, abundant, loved", it sends that energy out into the universe. Whether in thought or spoken word, it releases the power of co-creation and whatever is predominantly uttered after the 'I AM' is formed in the world of energy. Repeated utterances and dominant thoughts with emotion behind them, create stronger manifestations.

The I AM light and presence can be magnified and diminished within you. You can ignore it, thereby it stays a tiny spark (like a pilot light in an oven) and you can also ask God to pour the I AM presence energy and light into your physical body and aura with even more powerful Divine energy. Igniting that pilot light into a fully formed, body-sized flame to meet the light you just called in. The benefit in doing this, is by bringing in more Divine energy into your field, you feel more connected, calmer and confident.
I like to do this every morning, and even throughout the day if I remember to. Things seem to flow more when I do this. When you ask, visualize a white pillar of light coming down through you and surrounding you, directly into the Earth beneath you.

The Higher Self is part of the Soul

Our Higher Self is the consciousness part of our Soul. A very elevated consciousness that is aware of everything about us and our path, and has a constant connection to God and our Spiritual Team. Your Higher Self is an eternal energetic consciousness that knows all about your past lives, your present life, and has the highest perspective for your potential futures in this lifetime. Your Higher Self knows you the best and understands you without the ego mind interfering. But interfere the ego mind does!

You may ask, why aren't we operating from our Highest Self all the time since we have this incredible connection within us? Well, part of the human experience is having the ego mind. It's the part of ourselves responsible for keeping us alive and safe in the 3D world. The instinct to fight, flight or freeze when exposed to danger. In modern times, we grow up with the ego mind dominating, but many young children are still remembering aspects of their Spiritual selves before birth, are more in touch with their Higher Self and being in the moment, its all about their own needs and wants. They feel, touch, sense, see, experience with abandon! Unfortunately, some children born into abusive households may not have that aspect prominent as they're focusing solely on safety and survival. There are many resources available about childhood development from both the practical and Spiritual points of view if you'd like to learn more.

My point is, as we move through family, school, and societal expectations, our ego mind becomes more prominent and dominating as we move into adulthood. For many, by the time we're adults, we need to undo a lot of programming and belief systems and re-awaken and re-connect to our Highest Selves once again. Doing so helps us live our lives from a more intuitive and less stressful standpoint, as opposed to a panicky fearful one that resists change. Our ego, Bless it, just wants us safe and secure. So, keeping the status quo and not moving out of our comfort zones is where our ego likes to happily stay. But when you start to feel tiny nudges of restlessness or gentle twinges of something disturbing existing conditions, that's your Highest Self giving you little signals to correct, change, or take action for your highest good.

Where does the Higher Self reside exactly?

It's within you and above you as a bridge to the Spiritual realm. We have the power to completely dismiss our inner knowing and shut it out through distractions, obsessions, and focused attention only on the material world. But by actively connecting and communicating with our Higher Self, we can operate from this heart centred place of inner wisdom. Actively calling in your Higher Self and bringing that energy in, down into your physical body, where it really is its rightful place, does not disconnect that bridge to the Spiritual world, on the contrary it also brings the Spiritual world closer to you. The only thing really separating us from the Spiritual world is our physical body, for we are Spirit incarnated into a physical body.

Visualization to bring in your Higher Self

Close your eyes.

Just breathe for a few breaths feeling your physical body, be aware of it from the top of your head down to your toes.

Then, imagine your Higher Self is an energy consciousness resting just above the crown of your head, like a giant white ball. It's moving and rippling, like its breathing.

Say in your mind *"I call in my Higher Self to come deeper into my physical body now"* and then visualize that white ball melting into and filling your head and neck, going down into your torso and arms, filling you with white light, going further into both legs and feet, right until the toes.

See in your mind's eye your inner body glowing white with your Highest Self energy.

Then, direct your attention to your heart, see it glowing golden there, where your Higher Self has 'locked in'. Breathe in and out from your heart a few times and affirm *"I now operate from my Higher Self and I only speak my Highest Truth".*

I suggest doing this in the morning before you start your day and repeating as often as needed, especially if you feel frazzled or disconnected, or unbalanced.

Why have our Souls incarnated onto Earth?

This is a huge topic, with the well-touted question "why are we here?" asked throughout the ages. I have simplified it according to my knowledge and Spiritual guidance.

Before the physical incarnated (embodied in flesh, in human form), where God existed, there were different dimensions around him/her (I use these pronouns because God represents both dualities. More on God in Chapter 4) with a variety of etheric light Beings; Angels, Dragons, Unicorns, and Souls not yet incarnated into anything physical. These light Beings were all created by God, all Divine sparks from God's energy Source, that came into being because God is a creator. God created so that his/her creations could experience their God-like selves (that spark) within different circumstances and environments. Some more challenging than others in order to show these Divine sparks their power to overcome, learn, and evolve past the situation they're in. And because of collective consciousness, which is that we are ALL connected energetically – humans, animals, plants, minerals, extraterrestrials, and God him/herself. God experiences it all with us. He/She sends light and Beings to help each and every one of us, those who have faith, those who are unsure, and those who turn away from God. He/She never intervenes with the free will of any of his/her creation otherwise there would be no learning, no wisdom and no Divine realization gained. He/She wants us all to realize our own power, our own co-creating abilities, to realize that we are not alone.

Before Earth as we know it existed, our Souls were in the higher dimensions as Beings in various civilizations. These were very high vibration civilizations with peace, equality, transparency, love and a symbiotic relationship with all Beings of creation. Everyone had full use of their sixth sensory abilities and there was a great sense of connected community.

Until a few Beings started to feel that they could have more, deserved more, and wanted to be more powerful like God, so they abused the power they had which allowed the lower energies in and dropped the vibration immensely. Which is where we find Earth today. In the third dimension. This has been referred to as "the Fall" and "fallen angels". In fact, most humans incarnated now are all "fallen angels", and part of this Earth school and in the wheel of karma and reincarnation trying to get back to that original Source energy in the higher dimensions as evolved Souls.

"The Fall" doesn't mean that there's an individual that is evil that we can blame all tragedies on, but instead that this capacity for lower base human emotions lies within each human and can lead one down the path to greed, rivalry, hate, etc. and further away and separate from God and our own Higher Self. It's our free will choice and reaction to each situation and person in our lives that creates a hell or heaven on Earth for each one of us. Humans have created the reality that is shaped today. We must take full responsibility for our actions and rectify them. It is never too late.

There are however, lower and darker energies that do exist but we don't need to discuss that extensively, just be aware of it. This is a guide for the highest light filled path and vibrations. Light must, and always shall, prevail.

Some readers may find this a bit too religious and it may be triggering. I respect that and I don't need to convince you of the origin story, you need only to be aware of the energies and how to work with them.

What's the goal of our Soul?

Earth is a very intense school. The hardest one in the Universe.
Earth offers the most incredible learning experience in all the Universe, a unique and special place that can provide challenges that speed up our growing and awakening process. Our end goal and point of our Souls' progression is to move back to Source, to the highest and purest dimension. We do that through many incarnations on Earth where we experience Soul challenges and lessons that we agree to undertake with other people, or on our own.
Our true home is as a Soul in the Spiritual realm.
Our Souls can grow and evolve easier and faster from human incarnations than just staying in the Spiritual realm. Since the Spiritual

realm has many like minded high vibrational Souls, it's hard to learn and grow around them, because if everyone is on your wavelength, things flow along peacefully with no challenges or lessons. So, in a lower vibration, Earth, we really speed up our learning with the aim to evolve as a Soul and return back to the highest vibration of everything.

Now, we're not completely abandoned to figure this out on our own. We all have an incredible Spiritual team to help and guide us. While they cannot help us entirely avoid our Soul challenges and lessons, they can help us through them easier, and with a perspective that it's a learning experience, which helps us release the trauma of energetic imprints. Even though we are born with the Veil of Amnesia, forgetting our Spiritual selves, where we come from and our past lives, we do have our Guardian Angel who never leaves our side, our Higher Self and a myriad of other Spiritual helpers who are constantly talking to us and trying to guide us (more on them in Chapter 5). All these aides to help us realize our true self, find our purpose(s) and always intuit what is best for ourselves.

So, when we incarnate into a lifetime, our Soul has chosen this lifetime specifically. A planning has gone on before birth in the Spiritual realm, with our Angels and Guides, where they show us the challenges, and we agree because we want to grow and expand. Some Souls may join us for a part, or throughout our lives, and we usually have a past life with them and could have karmic ties binding us together, especially if it's a challenging relationship. Or you could be the challenging one to another Soul. Everyone is on their own path and has chosen that path.

Some Souls come to heal, observe, experience, and assist others. Most Souls come to clear the energy (the karma) and grow, and wake up to their true essence and love themselves unconditionally. If we do not clear the karma with forgiveness, love and compassion (the usual antidote), our Souls can choose to come back for another incarnation to try again to clear it.

So essentially, in this brief human incarnation, in order to evolve to the next Soul level, we should strive to;
- forgive ourselves and others
- release toxic anger and negative emotions and energy
- have compassion for ourselves and others
- treat others as we'd like to be treated
- enjoy life! It doesn't have to be all hardship and challenges. God still wants us to enjoy our lives, in whatever form that means for you. (This does not mean ingest and imbibe everything to the point of addictions, but to enjoy other aspects of life as well)

What happens after Physical Death?

Physical death is the transition of when the Soul departs from the physical body. The time of death within the lifetime is usually organized by the Soul before reincarnation. The cause of physical death may not always be detailed out, and sometimes if it's a sudden death the Soul may be confused and not realize it's dead. This is when the Soul is still largely influenced by the human identity and their Earthly life. They may stay connected to the body, or a home, an addiction, a partner, or become trapped between the realms as an Earthbound Spirit. Some of them intentionally cling to their Earth life and habits because of fear of what's beyond.
Which is usually a life review with their Guardian Angel and Guides, and some Souls don't want to see that or face how their actions affected others. The Soul review, which cannot be avoided

once crossed over into the light, is a review of whether challenges or lessons have been met and overcome, or avoided. Then they go through a Soul healing for a time, depending on their lives.

The important thing to note is that the Soul lives on. Physical death is just physical death of the body. The Soul, and its characteristics from its last Earth incarnation go to a different dimension. Some are eager to speak to the living, some go on for further Soul evolution or study in Spirit form, and after some time, some may reincarnate again on Earth. I am often asked during Mediumship sessions if a passed loved one is with another passed family member. For instance, do all married couples meet up, or children with their parents. It depends. Each Soul is on their own path with their own unique circumstances.

For Souls ready to pass over, a light, or some form of a light appropriate to them, appears from their Guardian Angel guiding them back to the light from which their Soul came. Sometimes there may be relatives or friends greeting the Soul, or Angels, which can make the transition easier for the Soul if it was a sudden death.

When a loved one transitions, we certainly feel grief and must allow that process to happen and then gradually come out of it knowing you will most likely meet your loved one again, for only their physical shell is gone and dead, their Soul lives eternally. Excessive mourning or grieving, not letting go, has an energetic effect on the Soul that passed and if strong enough, can hold it back on its evolution in the Spiritual realm.

And I certainly don't mean forget they ever existed! From my communication with passed loved ones, I've learnt they all seem to appreciate a flattering photo of themselves in your home, maybe a flower or plant nearby. Something that makes you smile in remembrance rather than cry with sadness. It may take time to get to that place in your grieving process but really, your passed loved ones like to see you happy and enjoying life.

Some Souls do enjoy communicating with the living via a Medium, or create signs as physical manifestations for their loved ones on Earth to know they are nearby and not gone. Not all Soul are able to manifest in the physical world, but they can sometimes do so with the help of the Angels. Even if they can't physically manifest something for you, oftentimes loved ones come to visit you as an energy.

Earthbound Spirits

These are Souls of people who have died. Some don't move on to their next Soul experience for a variety of reasons. It could be a sudden death and they're shocked, or they had Earth addictions and are still feeling a draw to this dimension. Some feel like they have unfinished business, or are afraid to move on to the next phase because they don't know what that is. They may linger in places they went to in life to try to talk to the living, most of whom can't hear them, and after a while they get lonely or depressed or may finally realize they have died. Often, people think cemeteries are creepy and full of ghosts, but really, not many hang out there, there's no life in a cemetery. The Earthbound Spirits are all over the place, often in places where they had addictions, (bars, nightclubs, restaurants), or even grocery stores or just on the street, on public transit, or in buildings. They get energy from the alive humans around them. Whatever their reason for lingering, we should always try and move them along as there is no benefit to them staying around us. They're only slowing down their own Soul progress. Some can clairvoyantly see them, or we may feel them as heavy energies which make us feel exhausted or perhaps get sudden cravings or emotions which are not ours. Children usually act the opposite and get very hyper and manic if one of these Spirits are within their aura. Mediums and highly sensitive people can help them move on, also with the help of the Angels, Ascended Masters, Dragons and their own Ancestors.

NDE - A Near-Death-Experience

This is defined as an aware and conscious, out-of-body experience occurring at the time of death or threatened possible death. Many have written of their experiences and no two are identical but some have similarities in what was seen or experienced, and all who write about their experience have come back to their physical body and life here. You can find a great deal more on this topic with the Near Death Experience Research Foundation or, I found this author's experience quite interesting; Eben Alexander

What is a Past Life and Reincarnation?

Our Souls are eternal, they've experienced all of our past lives and carry our karma and ancestral karma as energetic imprints from a variety of notable events. We consciously forget all these things when we're born into a new incarnation as part of the evolving and growing process of our Soul. So, it's an important practice to explore where we've come from, where we are now, and where we want to go without carrying these negative experiences forward.

It's likely that many past lives have been lived by your Soul if you're reading this book. It is possible that a Soul can incarnate into just one lifetime for a specific role and purpose, but for most, we've lived through many and usually with our current family members or friends and colleagues. We accrue Karma in each lifetime. After physical death, we go through a Soul review to decide whether we want to be reincarnated (born again into a new human experience) once more to resolve what we didn't in the past lifetime.

Our Souls reincarnate to resolve or complete unfinished business on Earth which wasn't cleared in a previous lifetime. As we can't Spiritually advance until we clear it up. Avoiding it will not do us any good. Including family. We have etheric cords with family to clear up usually as the first challenge, but it could also be the only challenge. But as I've mentioned, we're born with amnesia, forgetting all our past lives and the Spiritual realm from where we came. Then the many distractions on Earth often make us forget our Spiritual goals. You can see why Earth is such an intense school!

Our past lives are hidden so we can live in the here and now but sometimes experiencing a past life regression can provide insight, healing, and release, for current issues we're facing. I found this book very interesting regarding past lives; Many Lives, Many Masters, by Brian Weiss, M.D.

Each Soul does have the free will choice of whether to reincarnate again or not. They may choose to stay in the Spiritual realm for further study and learnings before reincarnating again, if ever. But usually, another lifetime on Earth provides faster progress. However, each Soul is on their very individual path in the journey back to the highest dimension.

What is Karma?

This is part of the Law of Cause and Effect. What we sow, we shall reap. It means you'll experience the same kind of things you've caused another person to experience. Karma is accrued in all of our lifetimes, and can be perceived as a boomerang of our own thoughts, words, and actions that come back to us. This gets stored in our bodies, genes and Soul if we don't take action to dissolve karmic effects, which is essentially the path of forgiveness, compassion and love.

Once incarnated as a human, we are in the cycle of karma, especially if we choose to have children. And we continue to be reincarnated as a human to overcome the lessons and challenges with the aim to stop the cycle of karma. Once you've incarnated as a human, you do not come back as an animal, insect or tree. It would make no sense as the karma accumulated can only be resolved as a human Soul learning and evolving. To come back as an animal for example, who knows only love and has no karma, is like having a lifetime stagnant. Can it work the other way? An animal coming back as a human? – No, animals don't accrue karma so to come back as a human would be a very long commitment on Earth school in order to eventually rid itself of the karmic burdens. Because in each new life, we accrue more karma unless we really live a high vibrational life, fully in a state of compassion, forgiveness and love so that if any karma is accrued it comes back to us faster (in the same lifetime) and we can resolve it faster rather than bringing it on into the next incarnation.

Ancestors and Genealogical Lineage

You are energetically connected to all of your past ancestors. The ones you may have met; aunts, uncles, grandparents. And also to the ones you don't know, stretching back through time and past incarnations. These little energetic spots in your timeline can carry a variety of characteristics and traits from past ancestors. For instance; lack mentality, persecution complexes, physical disorders, fears, a propensity for injuries and more. Some of their karma can also be carried within your DNA. This would be from karma they haven't come back to complete in another incarnation, or deeds that were just too overwhelming to complete in the lifetimes they had. These leave an imprint on their Souls, which have a lesser imprint on your Soul but are still present through the genealogical lines. When we heal ourselves and release our own triggers, we are healing the ancestral line all the way back through the timelines and they feel it and thank you for it.

Your Family in this Lifetime

As mentioned earlier, we make agreements with other Souls to incarnate together, for our own development, or for theirs. We've most likely already had past lives with them and this definitely applies to biological and adopted families. There are no coincidences. As a Soul before birth, we choose our parents, we are attracted to mothers and fathers of a similar vibration of our Soul challenge.

Our first teachers in life are our immediate family, indirectly, or directly through their examples. Often there is conditional love taught first – *"if you do this, mommy/daddy will love you"*, which is then what we learn. We are trained to crave their love, approval and acceptance. And they do their best, they follow on with how they were taught and brought up. But it's not entirely their job to do this, it's our job to learn to love, approve and accept ourselves. Think of this affirmation: *"It's not important what others think of me, it's only important what I think of myself."* Part of growing up is loving ourselves, if we can't do that, we can't love others. There's really no way around it. Otherwise, we seek and crave external validation of our worth and capacity to be loved.

So if there's anything we don't like in our parents, this trait is also in us. If a family member pushes our button, this is something reflecting back to us. This person, or people, are our teacher, our catalyst to change ourselves. At a Soul level, we have consciously selected a cast of characters as family to help us on our growth path. So taking a higher perspective to a troubling relationship and keeping this in mind can help you start to shift to forgiveness and compassion. It doesn't mean you have to be in a close relationship (unless that is the challenge), but holding grudges binds us to them, and if not resolved, it carries into future lives and our offspring. Only forgiveness can dissolve these ties.

It's also important to realize that we're not here to heal that person, or change them, this is their own life and path. We are here to heal the problem we have with that person. We need healing and positive energy to replace the toxic energy. There is no blame we should apply to our parents, no matter how horrific they may have been, instead we can thank them for giving the perfect environment of growth and awakening for ourselves. We can spend decades, or most of our adult life working on healing these relationships, considering the abuse that may take place between parents and child. The power often lies within us to end the negative pattern. For instance, someone may have been raised in a home that was emotionally cold and abusive in some form. That child can go on to apply the same cold and abusive home to their children, OR, they can decide to offer a completely different home environment of love, affection, support and warmth. That choice is how you can overcome a Soul challenge and end an ancestral family pattern.

Channeled Message from the Orange Dragon: "There has been a separation with the family units among humanity. The intent in the beginning was for your parents to birth you, to give you a physical avenue into this incarnation. Then, the goal was to either experience the Soul challenges and overcome them and learn the lessons which would give cause to your own Soul evolution. Becoming an independent fully formed Soul Being within your own physicality and with feet firmly established on your path forward. What has evolved is a mish mash of co-dependent relationships, control and manipulation of a child's path within a structured system without allowing their right brain, their feminine intuitive side to flourish and grow as they grow up while learning to balance with their left brain, their masculine organized side. Families were to live in communities of sharing, cooperation and while not exactly co-parenting, but in a somewhat traditional tribal system. As per the old adage 'it takes a village to raise a child'. These kinds of communities would establish and foster that sense of Oneness of all humanity. We all have the same Soul spark within us, the Divine spark. Which come from the same Source. It doesn't mean you lose all sense of individuality and uniqueness. Not at all. Everyone is unique and has their own purpose and path without the need for competition. But the plan was to be unique and be part of a great community. I use a metaphor for modern times. In a well playing sports team, each team member has their own particular skills they excel at, yet working together as a team brings their whole sum of greater value than their individual parts when working towards a common goal. Which in this case, is to score goals. What each individual team members responsibility is to ensure their own skills and fitness. Their flow, physically, emotionally, mentally and Spiritually. Then, to appreciate and understand the other team members strengths and how they can all work together like puzzle pieces fitting into slots to make the whole picture. That's a lot of metaphors but it is to understand the optimal paths.

*For it is not too late, humanity can change their ways and beliefs
with perseverance and understanding with open hearts."*

At this point of reading, you may start to realize how much responsibility we have in our lives regarding our holistic well-being.
We are the masters of our energy and have the power to shift the
energy through various means at our disposal. Everyone heals and
needs healing in a different way but with perseverance, dedication
and application, it can be achieved! The time required to heal may
not be overnight, but again even that is according to the individual
and their path. Life is a healing process.

Life Purpose

"What is my life purpose?" is a frequent question during my sessions
with clients and sometimes there isn't a very specific and definitive
answer as we'd like. As you've learnt, our Souls are on their own path
and trajectory and each of us have our own unique purposes. Often
more than one. It's not like everyone incarnates to be famous and
influential and change millions of peoples' lives. Sure, there are some
who incarnate for a role like that. But there are millions more who
incarnate for a variety of big and small reasons. There's a myriad of
purposes and paths each Soul is on, intertwined with other Souls,
coming in and out of lives for a reason, a season, or a lifetime. Also,
your purpose does not always mean your career or job. One does
not always generate income from their purpose.

The best thing we can do is figure out who we are, get in touch
with our inner self, understand what we love to do with passion
as well as realizing what our natural gifts and skills are. That could
mean undoing and dropping a lot of societal, family and cultural
conditioning. It takes courage and time, especially if you're already a

mature adult reading this. In addition to the self-exploration, asking your Higher Self and your Spiritual team to help you figure these things out, help you get on your path and stay on it, is a key part of the process. For instance, in a psychic reading you may ask about your life purpose and you will get an answer for sure. It may be a vague future potential, but most definitely advice on the next step you need to take. I wish it was a 10 year plan given with the end result! But this is part of our human experience and Soul path to discover ourselves, plus our free will choices can change so much.

I once heard Abraham talk about this for Esther Hicks (she channels a group of light beings named Abraham in front of hundreds of people). They said if they had told her when she was starting out that this is what the end result will be, she would have immediately put up resistance and denial saying 'oh no, I don't like, or want to do public speaking' and it would have stopped the flow. So sometimes it's better to just be aware, step by step, as our Spiritual team usually have far greater plans for us than we can imagine for ourselves.

Don't be discouraged though, it's never too late to get on your path and your team never abandons you.

Soulmates

We each have many Soulmates and not all are romantic ones. We often feel like we have a deep connection and affinity with these individuals. Before incarnation, we make agreements with other Souls to meet in the coming lifetime for various reasons. Not always for heavy lessons and challenges, but it could be to feel more love, receive an opportunity, or be a friend at a time when its most needed. Soulmates can be friends, lovers, marriage partners, business partners, colleagues, family. Your path may be to meet that one romantic Soulmate and you'll have a wonderful happy lifetime together or perhaps you'll have fewer years together for lessons and teachings and then part. But then other Soulmates come into your life later. It is very individual to the Soul involved. But a Soulmates role or entry into your life is never to fill a void or to make you feel better about yourself. That can only come from our own self-love, self-acceptance and self-appreciation.

Twin Flames

Twin flames are two halves of the same Soul. The same Soul split into two different physical bodies. It's unusual to have them incarnate together at the same time, unless it's for a greater worldwide purpose. With Soulmates, we are still teaching and learning and navigating our way through this lifetime. With a Twin Flame, there's nothing to learn or teach and therefore our Soul doesn't progress and evolve. So more often, one Twin Flame would stay in Spirit form, a guide, a member of your Spiritual team, to help the one that incarnates. Not everyone has a Twin Flame, some Souls do not split for their own reasons.

I personally don't feel it should be as exalted and romanticized as it is with people spending a lifetime looking for their Twin Flame or *the* Soulmate.

A more beneficial route would be to work on ourselves, healing, releasing, building up our own confidence and following our path with happiness. We then attract the same high vibrational, happy people into our lives just by being ourselves. But we can't attract these people who are a right match for us in with desperation or constant yearning, or negative self-talk. It's better to wait to be happy with the right person for us, than unhappy with the wrong one for us out of fear of being alone.

More about Souls and the Spirit Realm

If you'd like to learn more about Souls and the Spirit realm, there are numerous books on the topic. A few that I enjoyed are by Sylvia Browne, Dolores Cannon and Allan Kardec.

2 ▎

The Mental and Emotional
Soul Path

Our Energetic Systems

The Chakras

We have energy centres in our physical body and personal energy field, which receive and bring in Universal Life Force Energy as well as expel our own energy. Energy in this case, meaning our emotions, thoughts, words, and belief systems. These energy centres are also known as consciousness centres, but more commonly known as Chakras (the name comes from Eastern disciplines). There are seven main chakras running along the core of our body, as well as minor chakras throughout our torso and limbs and higher vibrational chakras within our auric field. These energy centres are each connected physically to organs, our nervous system, glands, our mental, emotional and spiritual states of being. The chakras absorb the Universal Life Force Energy, break it up, and send it to the physical body systems. In addition to the physical, the state of our chakras also greatly affect our mental and emotional inter communications.

Each of the seven major chakras spin with their opening on the front of the body as well as on the back of the body (see the image at the back of the book). They have their own seven layers that correspond to a layer in our auric field and all layers must be open for the energy to flow smoothly and unobstructed. The open end of a healthy balanced chakra in the first layer is about 6 inches diameter extending about 1 inch from the body. The chakras spin as vortexes, swirling like whirlpools, and they bring in energy as well as leak out energy if not careful. Each major and minor chakra allows energy to flow in and out. We're like sponges in the sea of energy around us. We experience this energy as feeling, seeing, hearing, sensing, intuiting or direct knowing. Empaths can feel this as an overwhelming flow of information and often have to close their energy or avoid places with large crowds. Most people process the energy surrounding them according to their current state of personal development.

The importance of opening and balancing the chakras throughout life is important as when they open, they increase the energy flow and the healthier we are. Many illnesses are caused by, or contributed to, by an imbalance of energy or a blocking of the flow of energy in our human system. A block or imbalance also distorts our consciousness and can affect our emotional and mental well-being.

If one chakra is out of balance, it affects the others. I suggest that a chakra clearing and balancing is a helpful additional treatment protocol for anyone suffering from a chronic or acute physical ailment. In order to treat the person as a whole we need to look at all imbalances, whether they're physical, mental, or emotional.

Young children are so close in time to when they were Soul beings without the physical incarnate yet, that their whole body emanates Soul energy, it's why they're completely in the present moment, focused on themselves. Their chakras are not yet fully developed when born, they're there, but much smaller and they develop as the child grows, starting with the root chakra, which is their first developed chakra – am I safe, secure, fed, warm, nourished it asks. As they grow into adulthood, the chakras develop and the Soul is being expressed through the chakras. And since the chakras allow our emotions and thoughts to express out into our aura, this is how our energy can become heavier and more burdened as we get older and experience more of life.

In the Chakra chart found at the back of this book, I've listed the seven core chakras located within our physical body, and the higher vibrational chakras along with their location, associated energy, organs, crystal and the Archangel and Dragon (more about them in Chapter 5) overseeing the chakra. I have not listed the colours as the colours can change depending on the state of being in the individual.

The higher vibrational chakras (stellar, soul star, causal, Dragon, navel, earth star) lie dormant for most, but when opened and awakened, bring so much more spiritual depth into one's life.

There are also numerous minor chakras, which are still energy points along the body, often coinciding with a Meridian line as well. At the end of the day, it's still ALL energy.

How to open and balance your Chakras

In Part Two, we'll cover the many modalities and tools that you can use to help open, clear, heal, and balance your chakras. I started my chakra maintenance when I learnt Reiki and continue to do it regularly to stay balanced. It's a continuous process as our chakras constantly fluctuate with our emotions, thoughts, words, actions and life experiences.

The Aura

The Aura is our invisible force field, an energy field surrounding the physical body like an egg, normally extending outwards a few feet but can expand or contract as well. It's a representation of our life force. Meditation, an energy healing session, or walking in nature are common aura expanders. For someone who is very physically ill or on the cusp of their transition, their aura will contract as their life force may not be radiating as strongly.

To feel your own energy in your aura, try this exercise; hold the palms of your hands facing each other about 10 inches apart. You will almost immediately feel some energy between your hands, perhaps as pressure, or a tingle. You can also practice by holding your hand a few inches above certain body parts. Maybe over that sore knee you may feel more tingly compared to the healthier knee. We are constantly and consistently radiating our energy outwards. This energy we radiate comes from our spiritual, mental, emotional and physical selves.

It's not just humans who have an aura. Animals, trees, rocks, flowers, insects also have one, as well as objects such as jewelry, pillows, furniture and cars. Although the inanimate objects have a large part of their energy made up of accumulated energy from the humans and/or animals that have handled or sat or slept on the objects. But the natural world vibrates with its own energy auras. Because of this, I recommend that if you buy second-hand of any kind, be sure to energetically cleanse them (tips in Chapter 8) before bringing them into your home as you'll also be bringing home the whole weight of energy with that object. Some could be good, some perhaps not so good.

These auras are all a part of the Universal Energy Field that we all exist within. The Universal Life Force Energy that surrounds us, and is a part of us.

But the aura is not just a shell that surrounds us, it's full of so many things that represent ourselves at that moment in time when looking at it. The state of our auras continually change in colour and density, based on our emotional, mental, physical and spiritual state. Everything we experience as a human we throw into our energy like it's a kitchen sink. Hoping the negative things get drained away if we just stamp them down below into the drain. But things never really disappear, they just get stamped deeper. Dormant for years until one day we're triggered by another person, circumstance or life event. Or, unresolved issues can sometimes manifest into a physical ailment.

Through our aura and all it contains, is how we interact energetically with the physical and spiritual worlds. So you can see how important it is to care for our holistic well-being!

This is why sometimes you can feel someone's 'vibe' when meeting them, or feel the energy of a room when walking into it. Everyone is emanating their thoughts, emotions and belief systems out from their aura. Empaths, and very sensitive and intuitive people, can easily tune into this energy floating around you, which is quite beneficial especially if they're assisting you during an energy healing session or psychic reading.

There are seven auric layers and each level holographically holds energy related to your life's story. From conception, until death. They're made up of vibrations, the subtle energy from your physical, mental, emotional and spiritual selves. The flow and movement of this energy throughout your body can have a major impact on your health and well-being.

Seven Energetic Bodies of the Aura

While I list the chakra that each layer is associated with, each chakra actually has a layer within each auric body. Humans are very multi layered and complex beings!

First Layer - Etheric Body

This layer extends ¼ to 2 inches from the physical body. It's the energy representing the physical body; muscles, tissues, bones, etc. The etheric body already surrounds an embryo as it develops and grows into a baby in the womb.

This is the densest layer and each following layer gets lighter in frequency as they move away from the physical body.

It is connected to the root chakra.

Practice Tip: Ask someone to stand against a white wall (preferably not wearing black), while you stand about 6 feet away, allow your gaze to relax and unfocus and let it fall on their shoulder, or around their head. After a little while, you may start to see a radiating energy, glow, or colour from their physical self. You can also practice with inanimate objects.

Second Layer - Emotional Body

The next layer is the emotional body and extends a little further outward from the physical body, from 1-3 inches. This layer is associated with our feelings and can be vibrantly full of colour or dark and murky depending on your mood. The colours come from the chakras.
It is connected to the sacral chakra.

Third Layer - Mental Body

This layer extends 3-8 inches from the body and is associated with our mental processes, our thoughts, ideas and belief systems. Sometimes a colour from the emotion felt in the emotional body is seen behind a certain thought or idea, making it more well-formed and stronger within the mental body. By focusing on these thought forms we enhance their effect on our lives. Habitual thoughts become even stronger and more powerful. This layer can be a strong yellow colour when a person is deep in thought, but this can change if the thoughts are very emotional and then the colours come from the layer below.
It is connected to the solar plexus chakra.

Fourth Layer - Astral Level

This layer extends outward ½-1 foot from the physical body and is our first connection to the Spiritual realm from the physical body. It's closely linked with the emotional body and can often represent the same colours but all with a tinge of higher vibrational love energy, so softer, more pastel colours. This is why ascended chakras (those radiating at a higher vibration) often change colours to a more pastel hue. A fully opened heart chakra is pink on the astral level.

Guided Meditations such as Raising your vibration with the Angels from my YouTube channel, bring in the highest Angelic energy into the chakras to help raise their vibration.

It is connected to the heart chakra.

Fifth Layer - Etheric Template Body

This layer extends from 1 ½ - 2 feet from the physical body and is the entire blueprint of the physical body and first etheric layer. It includes everything you've created to represent yourself on a physical level, such as your identity, personality and overall energy. It's how you express yourself to the world.

This is connected to the throat chakra.

Sixth Layer - Celestial Body

This is the layer that connects us to the Divine and extends about 2-2 ¾ feet from the physical body. It contains a powerful vibration. This is the emotional level of the spiritual realm and when we are truly and fully connected with the Divine, and see the light and love in everything that exists, we only feel unconditional love, joy and bliss. This spiritual bliss usually happens during deep meditation when the lower layers are quiet.

It is connected to the third eye chakra.

Seventh Layer - Causal Body

This is the final layer of the auric field and is the egg shaped 'shell' around our physical body and the other six layers. It can extend from 3-5 feet or more from the physical body depending on the activity of the person and it vibrates at the highest frequency. This is the mental level of the spiritual realm and when we bring our consciousness to this level, we understand and know we are one with the Divine and all around us. It's a very strong field and protects the auric energy fields like a shell protects a baby chick. It contains everything within it on a golden grid and contains your life plan in this incarnation.

I have also read various sources speaking about the Crystalline Light Body. From my guidance, this layer can be seen as being your Crystalline Light Body. It's your highest state of being, a higher dimensional state of consciousness still within a physical body.
Babies and some children naturally emit this light through their innocence and purity.
It is connected to the crown chakra.

The above auric layer information is provided from this book, Hands of Light, by Barbara Ann Brennan which I highly recommend if you'd like to read further about your energy fields.

In Chapter 8, I give a few tips on how to clear your Aura.

The Meridians

There is another energetic system within the body, connected to our holistic body and also used as a medium of healing; the Meridian System.

Meridians in the human body are energy (known as Qi, pronounced 'chee') pathways, super highways of energy that constantly flow within us. Blocks or stagnant flow can manifest as physical or emotional distress. If chakras are our energy centres, Meridians are the road map of energy flowing throughout all parts of the physical body. There are fourteen main Meridian lines, which are connected and paired with yin and yang organs for perfect balance.

Two of these main lines are called the Governing and Conception vessels and are the main rivers of the body's yin and yang energies. These run on the front and back vertical midline of the body. Their pathways are complete, being composed of an ascending energetic flow and a descending energetic flow. The duality of these two lines join at the head and the perineum, forming a complete circle of energetic current.

There are also Extraordinary Meridian lines not connected to an organ but assisting with circulation and flow of energy throughout the physical body. Within all these lines are the balance of yin and yang, and for the body to function properly, there must be balance between the two always.

What are Yin and Yang? They are balance. Two parts making a whole. You may have seen the symbol, a circle divided by a curved line; white (yang) on one side, and black (yin) on the other. Yin is night, moon, female, still, cool, feminine. Yang is sun, day, energy, male, hot, masculine. The balance between the two is extremely important, if one is weak, the other will be stronger.

Acupuncture, Accupressure, EFT, the Eden Method, and more, are all modalities working with the Meridian system of the human body.

That covers all the energy systems of our human selves. You can see how many layers and facets make up who we are. What else can have a strong effect on our energies?

The Energy of Strong Emotions

Energetic Cords

Everything is energy. So it stands to reason that every substantial interaction we have with another person, whether it be written, on the phone or computer screen, face to face, or even just thinking of a person with a strong emotion creates an energetic cord between you and that person.

We develop energetic cords with everyone we speak with, especially if there's a lot of strong emotion behind the words. For instance, there are core family cords between parent and child that cannot be cut but can be cleaned, and in a romantic relationship, there are cords of love between heart chakras. When people are in a romantic relationship, especially a long one, cords develop between the two of them from many chakras (not just the heart) and many layers, and if that relationship ends, it's very important to remove the cords from both sides to help the grief and healing process and allow each other to move on.

As well, energy is transferred during sexual intimacy. A cord can develop from the root chakra but you can also absorb energetic imprints on various other parts of the body. For instance, heavy energy can lodge in the throat from the other person after oral sex.

So, it's a good practice to be very mindful of who you share your energy with intimately. And if it's a fleeting meet up, then don't forget to energetically cut cords and cleanse yourself afterwards (see how in Chapter 8).

People can also project their own energy outwards unconsciously if feeling especially sad, angry, or just plain irritable which we can un-intentionally pick up in our own auras. We must be very discerning to recognize what is our energy and what isn't. I've been grocery shopping and come back in a very low and irritable mood for no particular reason, so I did a process to energetically cleanse myself, and after 30 minutes or so I felt better and realized those emotions weren't me, it was energy I picked up. Energetic protection before-hand helps too of course, but if you're pulled out of your centred state for even a moment, (for instance, annoyance at other drivers, or at someone who was rude to you), you can so quickly attract even more of that energy. The ideal is going out of the house with a mindfulness of white light shining around you and being within your space, get your things done and be pleasant with the people you encounter, regardless of their mood, and leave. It does take a lot of focus to do that, and if you're shopping with someone, like your children who you have to keep an eye on, it's almost impossible. So, energetic cleansing once home, or at the end of the day, is a very good practice (Tips in Chapter 8).

Energetic Imprints
Very emotional or traumatic interactions leave an energetic imprint on us and our surroundings too.

The imprint is the memory of the energies that produce it and are found in the area where they were created, such as a location, a person, or on objects. You may feel these imprints in your own energy field and possibly take some of it away with you, burdening you with heavy energies that are not your own.

For instance, locations of horrific traffic accidents often have this imprint still there, or ancient trauma on the land (of people that were forcibly removed, tortured, killed). It's a good idea to energeti-cally clear the land before any new builds, or even renovations. The land emanates an imprint, some more subtle than others, but it will definitely affect the structure built on top of it.
This is why many homes, businesses, stores, places of worship, hos-pitals, schools, etc., have a feeling or vibe that is felt when you walk in. A home where there are a lot of arguments and crying will feel

heavy and oppressive, homes with a lot of joy and laughter will feel lighter. An office space that all the employees hate to be in will reflect that energy, whereas a place with a good workplace camaraderie will also be felt. Hospitals can have a very heavy energy due to the physically ill patients and their fears, but also the families and friends who visit and are full of worry. There may also be a lot of earthbound spirits in hospitals who may have not realized they passed just yet!

Even TV shows and movies can emanate energy into the space it's being watched in. First, it affects our personal energies as we absorb it into our eyes, mind, and in some cases, heart. And I've seen some darker topic documentaries bring in that smoky dark energy from the TV and sit in front of it. It doesn't mean you can't watch what you like, but these are all good reasons to clear your energy and the energy of your home regularly (Chapter 8). And definitely when you move into a new place, to get rid of the energy from previous residents which may still be lingering.

I had a teacher who taught us to read energetic imprints at sacred sites. We were in Ephesus, Turkey visiting various ancient temples and ruins. We sat down and focused on our breathing, moving into a calm and centred state, with palms open and out, sensing the energetic energy of the place. Some of us received flashes of visuals, some got a knowing. However it was received, there were still energetic imprints there thousands of years later. For myself, in an amphitheatre type of place, I saw a visual of the horse activities that took place there. It was just a flash, but there. The power of energy is phenomenal and there is so much to sense and see all around us.

You can also try this with your local trees. Select a large, rather old one and place your palm on its trunk and first send love or blessings to the tree and then ask it to share its story with you, or it's wisdom with you. Close your eyes and just allow the information to come in. Again, it may be visual, a knowing, a word, everyone receives differently and according to their state of being. I don't always get visuals, once I put my hand on a very tall older tree on a hiking trail and I just got the word 'steady', and then 'strong', a feeling that his roots ran deep and far.

Energetic imprints on people are usually traumatic experiences still contained within the auric layers and energy of a person, or an over-whelming depression or grief emanates as someone's energy and can imprint on others. This can go as far back as abuse from childhood or a recent divorce. Our cells, our bodies, our energy remember and contain every single thing that has happened to us, been said to us, and been done to us.

Imprints on objects such as clothing, jewelry, cars, phones, kitchen appliances, will take on the energetic imprint of the previous owner(s) and for new items, the energy of where they came from and the transport they experienced. So, it's a good practice to ener-getically cleanse (Chapter 8) everything you bring into your home. I like to clear all items I bring in my house, including groceries. I sometimes use White Sage, or I'll ask the fire Dragons to clear.

Energetic Attachments

These can either be Earthbound Spirits that cling onto our energy because they are attracted to our Life Force Energy (something they no longer have). As discussed earlier, if you have one of these in your energy field, you may feel exhausted, drained, or have inexplicable cravings for certain things. Young children often react the opposite, becoming more hyper with an attachment. Usually asking an intuitive, or energy practitioner to help move these spirits along is the best way. But with sharpening your own intuitive senses, you can also learn how to help these stuck spirits go to the light.

The other type of attachment is an energy blob, it could be an energy you picked up or passed through. You'd feel similar effects with a blob, or just feel not quite right more than exhausted. Either way, the best thing is to remove all energy that is not your own on a daily basis. I usually call in Archangel Michael of the Highest Light or the Fire Dragons to clear but you can utilize whatever resonates with you. (Chapter 8).

Anger and Unforgiving

These are two of the strongest emotions that keep us weighed down and unable to let go and move forward. But we need to have compassion for ourselves at the time it takes to heal and release. It may have taken decades for the trauma and emotion to build up (possibly past lives as well), so it'll take time to heal. A lot of it is a mind shift, which automatically affects your energy. The first step is clearing the energetic impact, the trauma, from your body, and then it's a process in re-programming your mind by being mindful of your reactions. Maintaining a sense of detachment so that you are not reacting, bothered, hurt, affected by the person, event, trauma. Easier said than done I know! It's a constant vigilance of your thoughts, emotions, self-talk and actions. Being mindful in the moment is key. Not thinking about the past, and replaying what happened and how horrible that person is, or the future, or what might happen in the future or revenge. Please don't be discouraged by this prospect, with self-work and self-awareness, perseverance, and help from other professionals, and practitioners, we can heal, and we can become more sure of who we are and what we will accept.

The goal is to forgive and thereby release a lot of toxic emotions rooted in unforgiving like anger, resentment, shame, hurt, loss of control. It doesn't condone what was done, but it releases you from the toxicity and helps you move on.

Which brings me to the power of forgiveness. When I first started my journey, I was thinking, no way could I be so forgiving and forgetting. It's one of the hardest things to accomplish in our human lives (at least for those as stubborn as myself!). Because we have our strong sense of ego, and we've been raised in a society of victim vs abuser, with someone always to blame and punish. Blaming someone else for your problems or situation places your power within their hands. As essentially, you're saying I can never be happy because that person did this to me, or I'm so unlucky I never got a break. Remember the I AM statements? Watch what you say as it attracts more of the same.

I once read a children's book by Neale Donald Walsch about forgiveness which really helped me see the whole concept from a different and certainly higher perspective. It was a story about little souls in their realm of Heaven. They were excited at a new adventure starting soon, for they were about to incarnate into human physical bodies on Earth. Their purpose to incarnate was to experience everything and one of the things the little soul wanted to experience was to be forgiving. Now there's a lot of chances to forgive in our lifetimes, from something as small as forgiving someone who cheated us out of a few dollars, or to something far bigger like someone who limited our freedom, or abused us. Another little soul in heaven approached the first little soul and said "I will incarnate with you and give you the opportunity to forgive me for something I will do to harm you." And the first little soul said "but what on earth could you do to harm me, you are as light and love filled as me!" And the second soul said, "yes, so I volunteer to lower my light and vibration to such a low and dense level so that I could inflict harm against you. It may be verbal, or physical, or some other way. I will do this for you so that you can experience the act of forgiveness. By forgiving, this is a way of expressing love. And love is really all that is. We are the religion of love." Oh my said the first little soul, "what a sacrifice, thank you!" "But remember," said the second soul, "if you don't forgive me during this incarnation, we will go back lifetime and lifetime to repeat this pattern until you learn and act upon this and forgive me. Since you're going to forget this conversation and everything about Heaven as soon as you're born, this will be a challenge. But boy will we both rejoice once we're back here!"

I wish I could tell you the name of that book, I don't remember, but what's interesting is that my Guides brought that book to my attention in a hotel lobby in a remote area in the mountains where I had sat in an armchair for only a few minutes as I waited. (It was on a shelf next to the chair). It was clearly a message I needed to hear in that moment. This is just one example of how the Universe speaks to us constantly.

In forgiving someone who's hurt you, you don't have to love them, or feel love for them, or have a relationship with them. Just the act of forgiveness is the love you're extending. And mostly for yourself, bringing your power and control back to yourself, not in anyone else's hands. Not letting your past or story define you. It happened, see what there was to learn from it, forgive, and move on. If they're still in your life, that's where the boundaries come in. It's a process for sure. Remember to nurture yourself and forgive yourself throughout the process. We do the best we can.

Oftentimes, those difficult people we find in our lives are usually disconnected from themselves, projecting their dissatisfaction onto others. I'm not excusing anyone's behaviour but it's best to try not to take anything personally, even if this person may seem to have a vendetta against you. Always ground, protect and clear yourself before and after interactions but also send them Angels, you can visualize them being surrounded by white light and Angels. Sending back negative energy will only make it worse. You don't have to verbally say anything or treat them differently, but privately send them Angels. That way you don't set yourself up in a mire of negative energy swirling around you. And you won't react, whereas often people say or do things in order to get a reaction. Of course, if someone is abusing you, please get the necessary human help, as energy work and Angels can help, but sometimes it's a case where you, or someone else, may need to be removed from the situation.
This is a good book, The Four Agreements, by Don Miguel Ruiz that elaborates on not taking things personally.

The Power of Positive Emotions
It's not all doom and gloom though! It goes both ways, positive, uplifting and joyful energy is also contagious. Love, joy and humour spread like wildfire among us as well. If we all reacted to life's situations with these characteristics, the world would feel like a very different place right now.

We have the power and capability to emanate positive and loving emotions, thoughts, words and belief systems into the world around us. When we feel unconditional love and compassion, it automatically opens our heart chakras wider, allowing that love to flow in our fields. This is why pets are such great healers, they only offer unconditional love to us. The aggressive pets are sadly learned behaviours, as at their soul level, animals have open hearts ready to love unconditionally.

Feeling this love and compassion for fellow humans, whether family, partners, friends is an optimal place to be, but first and foremost feel it for yourself and expect it only from yourself. This will give you a lot more freedom than relying on external sources to make you feel better. Of course, it's wonderful to be loved and cared for by others, but it needs to start with us. Self-love, it's not just a catchphrase. We are so trained to compare ourselves to others, be concerned with what people think of us, find lack or judgment in our appearances and personalities, that it all overshadows our confidence and can make us live a large part of our lives being someone and doing things for other people.

Self-love is a belief that you are the most wonderful person on the planet and those who don't agree, well, it's not your concern. You prioritize yourself first and carefully cultivate and maintain your physical, mental, emotional, and spiritual well-being. It sounds like conceit and selfishness but it's really not. By caring for ourselves first, we can better help others from a happier and centred place. It's like they tell you on airplanes, in case of emergency, put your own oxygen mask on first before you put it on a dependent. Self-love is also being discerning on who and what you spend your time with.

Here are a few tips to help you practice self-love and build up your confidence. It's a process so please be gentle with yourself and forgive yourself if you stumble. You're undoing years of programming and conditioning so be patient with yourself.

Self-love Tips:

- Don't compare yourself to others. You are unique and on your own path.
- Try to care less about others opinions. Follow your own intuition on what's right for you.
- Forgive yourself if you make mistakes.
- Remember that your value is not in how your body or face looks.
- Set boundaries. Decide what you will and won't accept in all situations and relationships.
- Be mindful in your daily routine. What are you doing because you enjoy it, and not to make others happy.
- Practice being in touch with your Higher Self each day. Your Higher Self is totally in love with you and thinks you're the greatest.

Gratitude

How we view the world and our circumstances also contributes to our energetic well-being. Many have written about the power of gratitude. Being thankful for what you have, and even for what you don't have yet, but are manifesting, brings in a lot of the same positive energy of blessings. You could maintain a gratitude journal and write 3 things every day that you're grateful for, or when you wake up in the morning, mentally think of 3 things you're grateful for and give thanks for these things. To God, to the Universe, to your Spiritual team, yourself, whatever resonates with you.

Even if you're struggling financially, and cannot imagine where that money to pay rent, mortgage or groceries will come from, visualize you have it, *feel* the freedom and how relaxing that feels, and *thank* the Universe for providing you with this money. You're still living your life, taking action, but you're also expecting this money to come in, despite not knowing from where or how.

I remember a teacher I had telling us that when you have money, and you're not worried about it, that's how you attract more. There's no fear or desperation behind the requests, it's like being at a restaurant and you've just finished a big meal, you're sated and happy. You order dessert, not because you need it, because it would be a nice finisher. Not a big deal if they tell you they're sold out. You're not desperate to eat that dessert because you're hungry. I know, this is a difficult mindset when you're struggling and very worried and it requires a lot of mindfulness and 'fake it till you make it' attitude. The anguish of striving for something you desperately need causes its own resistance and less than positive energy spiral.

You can read further on the importance of your mindset from these authors; Napoleon Hill (Think and Grow Rich), Wayne Dyer, Louise Hay, Dr. Joe Dispenza, and Esther Hicks to name just a few.

Collective Consciousness
You now know how much responsibility we all have in cultivating and maintaining our optimal state of well-being, and just by taking care of that, we each have a direct impact on the planet and world we live in.

Everything in life is consciousness expressing itself in form, colour, fragrance and sound. We express it through our thoughts, speech, written words, actions, and emotions. The natural world and animals communicate their own consciousness into our world. And everything we're feeling, thinking, sensing, and doing is also being expressed into the world around us. Affecting others, and others affecting us. The environments we live, work and spend most of our time in, make an impact on our well-being. We live and move within an energetic soup of energy that we co-create and affects our lives.

All of life also shares the Divine spark. We all have that energy within us which came from the same Source. Whether you believe in a Higher Power or not, it's there. Like crumbs from the same giant cookie. Because of this, our Soul is connected with every other Soul on the planet. On a very subtle level, we feel what the majority are feeling.

On the negative side of the power of the collective consciousness, it's the cause of widespread panic, or mass hysteria within a large group when something alarming happens like a shooting or other aggression. The fear that spreads like wildfire in a traumatic event, the crowd picking up on the strongest emotion which is usually underlying fear. Hatred and rage come from fear.

The music festival Woodstock '99 had examples of crowd hysteria spreading throughout and causing a lot of abhorrent incidents. Now I'm not saying we can just absolve responsibility and say 'the crowd made me do it'. We're still fully responsible for our own actions, but my point is that the power and energy of a crowd can most certainly influence our own energies so let's use that power for good!

We can also feel immense joy, pride and celebration from a large group. Look at the energy generated from fans of a winning sports team. We saw this here in Canada when the basketball team, the Toronto Raptors, won their first NBA Championship in 2019, and more than a million took to the streets for the victory parade. I'm not a sports follower by any means and yet I found myself tearing up when I saw photos and videos of the energy that day, that delight and happiness everywhere. Because that joy is contagious, and who wouldn't want to be part of such joy and happiness?

Mass meditations are another powerful practice to shift energy in the world. When large groups of people gather together to meditate it creates ripple effects of peace in the surrounding environment. Imagine if large groups of people did it in every city of the world, at the exact same time, and how that peace would have an effect. Group meditations create a synergy of energy for a common goal, peace for instance. So when we all meditate together, the collective consciousness raises the vibration around the globe.
You can google the 'benefits of mass meditation' to read more about the studies done on it.

This act of humans working together for a collective goal and achieving that goal, or to provide a service or help to others, is one of the core facets of being human on this Earth right now. We are meant to work together, to be together, to have a sense of community, well, not just a sense, but BE the community. The incredible power wielded by many with a common goal and intention is phenomenal, with such a focused and determined lot of people, anything can be achieved and created. While society and the modern world has fostered and taught people to be the best, above all others, to win above all others, to do things just for oneself and one's own family, means we have for the most part lost this collective power. In history, the wise men and women, (often called witches and warlocks) found strength in a coven of many. It did not negate their own individuality, but enhanced it.

Sometimes human egos get in the way of a true and honest solidarity. That can be overcome when humans realize everyone has their own unique path and unique abilities to foster and offer the world. There is no need for competition. When one is in alignment with their Higher Self and the Divine, everything flows in accordance. There is no need to separate and divide. It only separates you from your true purpose. An analogy – when one battery is used to power a light, the light is powered yes but faintly. When 100 batteries are used to power a light, the light shines strong and bright and can be seen from far greater ranges than the first light. This is the power of the collective consciousness. Our energies towards a common intention are a driving force in the Universe and unavoidable by the universal law of attraction. We are co-creators. Let us be mindful of what we are creating with our energies.

Energetic Hygiene

That was a lot of information you just read, I know. The takeaway from this is that our lives and the world could be more peaceful and happier with mindfulness of our own energies and what we emanate into our surroundings. Mindful and discerning on how we spend our time and attention, and taking the time to daily cleanse and protect our energy. But also processing and releasing emotional baggage, toxic emotions and burdensome energy that we're carrying. We have to heal ourselves first. Just by doing that, our light shines brighter in the world, affecting others positively.

I offer some practical information in Part Two on methods to do this. You can select the ones that resonate with you, and that you have the time for. If you really want to start new habits and get on a higher vibrational path, I have a 21 day program for you to follow in Chapter 9.

At the end of this book, you can find image representations of our energetic bodies.

3

The Physical Self

Physical Body Systems

After exploring the energetic facets of ourselves, and what an incredible part of us they are, there's also the physical components of the human that comprises our holistic self. It's often our only focus! There are plenty of resources about nutrition, anatomy, exercise, and medical information so I'll only briefly cover our body systems and then focus on the physical aspects that are sometimes ignored.

Human Body Systems

Skeletal System - All of your bones.

Nervous System - Your nerves extending from your spinal cord and brain to every part of your body.

Muscular System - All of your muscles, tendons, ligaments.

Circulatory System - Your heart pumping, blood flow.

Respiratory System - Your breathing.

Lymphatic System - Your immune system, helps you fight off illness and protects you.

Endocrine System - All of your glands and hormones.

Digestive System - How your body processes the food and drink you ingest, nourishing, and then expelling waste via the anus.

Urinary System - Filtration of blood, expelling waste via urine.

Reproductive System - Your genitals which assist in reproduction, different in males and females.

Integumentary System - Your body's outer layer, your skin, hair, nails.

To refresh and boost your physical systems, you can listen to: Boost your Immune System Meditation on my YouTube channel, and also available on Spotify, Apple PodCasts, and Podbean.

Our Brainwaves

The human brain has billions of neurons (information messengers), and each neuron connects to other neurons, all very intertwined with each other. Communication between them happens through electrical impulses and chemical signals to transmit information to different areas of the brain and the nervous system. When a network of neurons are activated, they produce synchronized electrical pulses (like a rippling ocean wave), and this electrical activity is a brainwave. This is what's measured by an EEG (electroencephalograph). An EEG is one way to measure the electrical activity of our brain via electrical impulses which are active all the time, even while sleeping.

The results are usually described in terms of frequency bands. The rate of vibration or movement of the brainwaves per second, is measured as hertz.

These are the different measurements of human brainwaves and the state of being when in that vibration:

Gamma – greater than 30 Hz – Heightened perception

Beta – 13-30 Hz – Awake, normal alert consciousness

Alpha – 8-12 Hz – Physically and mentally relaxed, awake but drowsy, daydreaming

Theta – 4-8 Hz – Reduced consciousness, deep meditation, dreams, light sleep, imagination

Delta – less than 4 Hz - Deep (dreamless) sleep, loss of bodily awareness

Children are predominantly operating on different brainwaves than adults. In the womb and the first year of life, the baby is usually in the Delta waves, its why babies sleep a lot. In adults, we're in this state during our deepest sleep. From infancy until about 7 years old (although I've read some studies until 13 years old), a child's primary brain wave is in Theta, the imagination state. A time when their imagination runs wild, but also when they absorb all they hear. This state is highly programmable for this is the state adults are in during hypnosis to heal trauma or change belief systems, when information can be downloaded into the subconscious mind.

Children in this age range are like sponges, soaking up all they hear, see, and sense directly into their subconscious but without the ability to consciously evaluate the information as it's being down-loaded. For example, a criticism such as "you don't deserve that" or "you are bad" is not processed to understand the positive logic behind the negative critique in that instance. It's a deeper download of saying they are unworthy. Thus, it's very important to be conscious of what is being said to children and within their listening and visual distance.

Why is knowing about our brainwaves important?

The Planet Earth also has its own pulsating frequency and affects us too. Different frequencies have both positive and negative effects on the human body, and this can be further explained with the **Schumann Resonance.** in 1952, German physicist Winfried Otto Schumann documented the electromagnetic resonances between the Earth's surface and the ionosphere (the electrically charged part of the Earth's atmosphere). Within this pocket, the electromagnetic waves, originating from lightening discharges, resonated around a frequency of 7.83Hz. He surmised that this low frequency was the Earth's heartbeat. His research was later taken further by others who discovered that the Schumann Resonance match various levels of human brain activity when comparing EEG recordings with the Earth's electromagnetic fields. We are very much affected by our surroundings and environment, just as we affect the same on a mass scale.

The Earth's heartbeat at its base 7.83 Hz, is the Alpha/Theta state in our human brain, the relaxed, dreamy, sleepy state. A time of naturally occurring cell regeneration and healing. This explains why Earthing and Forest Bathing, or simply being in nature is such a healing balm for us. To compare, the things which power our cell phones, Wifi, TV and radios are in the **GHz**, quite a great deal more than what the Earth and our own brains radiate naturally and can contribute to a person feeling stressed, anxious, uneasy or have poor sleep among all these electromagnetic frequencies (EMF) in the air around us at all times, especially in congested places. I suggest a few tools in a 8 to help protect against excessive EMF radiation.

Water in the Human Body

This is not new information but important enough to mention. A healthy adult human body contains over 70% water, although this number varies with age. Most of this is within our cells and organs. The image at the back of the book shows how much water is within each major organ in the human body. It's a good practice to hydrate and drink enough water throughout your day to ensure optimal function of your body systems.

And equally important, the water within us also reacts at a cellular level to what we listen to. The physical element of water is affected by the energy we absorb. It's subtle, and likely won't make an effect until after extended listening, but it does affect us. You can google and read further about the interesting water experiments undertaken by Dr. Masaru Emoto who exposed water to positive and uplifting words and songs, as well as negative and derogatory words and songs. He compared the results as frozen water crystals, with the positive words creating beautiful designs within the water and the negatively exposed water becoming more dark and chaotic looking. Imagine what the types of music or words spoken to us could be doing to the water in our bodies!

Our Senses

Our five senses of Touch, Taste, Sight, Hear, and Smell are very well known and documented. We all know when we're feeling something by touching it, tasting something on our tongue, seeing with our physical sight with open eyes, hearing a song, or words, or various sounds around us, or smelling food, perfume, manure, or freshly cut grass. For most, these are senses we've grown up with, that were developed and understood more as we matured. We mostly sense our tangible world with these sensations.

But less discussed and acknowledged is our Sixth Sense - Our Intuition. This is our power of perception beyond the tangible world. It's the ability to just know something without any proof. It's feeling the energy within, around us, with other people, situations and places. The modern world places very little importance on this sense, and does not encourage children and parents to help their children tune into this sense, or develop it further. Those who do actively use it; empaths, psychics, energy healers, to name a few, are often viewed with skepticism and ridiculed. However, artists, writers, those who produce or work in the creative arts, are also tapping into their intuitive power. Oftentimes subconsciously channeling it into their work. Who is channeling this information to us? Ourselves. It's coming from that Soul being at our core, our Higher Self that has the highest perspective and overview of our lives. We are highly sensory beings, and as we've already discussed, made up of a great deal of energy that is constantly and consistently interacting with the world around us. Many people do it unconsciously and then might wonder why they're feeling so low or tired. Some are aware of the vibrational 'soup' around us and are diligent and mindful in their energetic hygiene practices and very discerning at what they expose themselves to. We only need to learn to tune in to our intuition, so we can get used to discerning what is that inner guiding high vibrational guidance and what is our ego, or negative belief systems, or other people's imprints. Imagine your body is a radio station that just needs a fine tuning to your inner voice. And that inner voice is connected to the entire Spiritual realm of help available to us which we'll discuss in Chapter 5.

Everyone feels their intuition, or gut instinct, in a way that's personal to them. For instance, some feel it as a pinch in the stomach area when something doesn't feel right, or an expansiveness and joy in the same area when they feel a good vibe or energy. Some feel tingles, or hear words, or get flashes of colours in their minds eye, or see shapes and masses with their physical sight. There's no right or wrong way to feel your intuition. And we ALL have this sixth sense. If you're not already tapped into it, (and that's okay, a lot can block our natural gifts. Children often act on instinct until they're told something is wrong or they'll receive punishment for it and then they start to inhibit themselves out of fear. Just an example of how we can bury our sixth sense from a young age!) you can develop it like a muscle with practice, intention, and perseverance. And once you do, the effort is well worth it. Imagine always making the right choice for yourself, taking the best path, or avoiding danger that is possible to be avoided. Trusting in your choices that the job, partner, home, vacation you chose is for your highest good.

4

The Universe Around Us

God

In the beginning, there was the Source of all that is. The Creator of the Universe. This is a conscious, omnipresent and omniscient energy comprised of Love. I refer to this Source as God, who has traditionally been depicted as a man in literature and artwork. However, God is both male and female energies, a Mother God and a Father God representing the duality in the Universe.

God created all the planets, minerals, animals, human beings and all the other beings in the Universe. We exist in this range of energy streams coming from the Source, God. These are a multi-dimensional range of energy, frequency and vibrations that are the basis of all there is and that gives us life. Our whole existence is just one energy manifesting itself in many different ways.

You may be a believer, or not. Or the talk of God may be a triggering topic. I'm not here to convince you, or make you a believer. Feel free to skip this part if you prefer.

But I would be remiss if I did not talk about God as part of Our Path. He/she is a huge part of it, really, the whole part of it.

Growing up, I was sent to Catholic schools as my parents thought they had a higher moral code and conduct. Well, that belief was mistaken but the teachers tried their best. I'm a non-practicing Catholic now, but I'm more spiritual and connected to God than I've ever been in my life.

God has also been referred to as Source, Spirit, All That Is, Supreme Being, The Creator, Divine Love, Holy Spirit, Universal Life Force, The Almighty, Heavenly Father, Absolute Being, The Alpha and Omega, I AM, Life, Omnipresence, Stream of Being, Primordial Stream, Spirit, All Intelligence, Light Ether, Eternal Spirit, Eternal Now, All Unity, All Communication, Consciousness, All Harmony, Eternal Being. There are likely even more names for God than I list here, and I respect all belief systems. Ultimately, all are referring to a Higher Power that we are eternally connected to.

Religion

(I do not speak on behalf of all religions here, only the one I grew up with.)

God's religion is Love.

He/she does not forbid, nor have human emotions of anger and vengeance, those stories are written by humans as religious dogma. The Christian Bible itself was written and put together by humans, translated, and interpreted over many different ages and according to the then current beliefs and aims of the clergy at that time. Perhaps some original content (by which I mean actual channeled wisdom from God) is still in there but I feel a large part of it has been adjusted.

Before the widespread use of the Bible, humans made offerings and requests in gratitude to God or Gods, an energy perceived as a greater power than their own. As seen by the weather, animals, and abundant nature. The offerings were minimal and symbolic, flowers, an herb, some food, gratitude, and respect were the core emotions. An honest and symbiotic relationship where humans worked with the cycles of nature, seasons, and animals. Not taking more than they needed, and never decimating a crop or animal for their own needs. They communed with the Nature kingdom for the best practices. (Findhorn Foundation is a modern day (1960's) example of working with the energies on how to grow food to feed the founders in a barren land. So, this skill is not lost to us.)

Unfortunately, the practice went downhill later on, when humans created more and more elaborate offerings, animal and human sacrifices and the clergy in charge of the temples and churches perpetuated this and ruled by fear and control. In today's world, we find the media and governments have taken over from the churches to rule by fear and control.

God never desired sacrificial offerings. The power of genuine gratitude, respect, and love is far more powerful. The idea that a human cannot commune or have no direct connection with God without an intermediary like a clergy member is one of the worst beliefs that was taught. God doesn't need a middleman to communicate to you, nor do you have to go to a special building to talk to him/her. When you think, when you ask, when you pray, what you feel, is also heard and felt by God. There is no separation.

As we've discussed, we all have a Divine spark within us and a Soul that came from God's energy, and therefore we ALL have the ability to connect and commune with God. Our Higher Self is in constant connection with God and the Spiritual realm.

You don't need to worship God within religious dogma in this lifetime in order to continue on your path. But of course, if you find comfort in being part of a congregation, then do what feels right for you.

For me, God is in my heart, a part of me, I am a part of him/her, he/she is around me, within nature, within each fellow human, animal, insect, all of creation. With every high vibrational spiritual Being I call upon, I know they come from and act for God. I don't follow any rules or dogma, I just try to act with love and compassion each day, treating others as I'd like to be treated. I'm not perfect, I make mistakes too and sometimes act with ego and fear, but am mindful to catch myself before I spiral too far. We all do the best we can.

My point is, that you have immense power within yourself to connect and commune with God. It's an individual connection and does not need an external party to help.

My intention is not to detach anyone from their faith or congregation, I just want you to be aware that your connection with God is internal and personal. You are your own sovereign power with a loving and supportive Higher Power within you and around you, always loving, helping, and accepting you.

The following examples were given to me by my Guides when I was pondering over this chapter. To show me how things may have changed since the original messages were given.

For instance, do you ever wonder why so many doctrines require head coverings? Mostly from women, sometimes from men. My

Guides advised me that this practice is not required by God. Our Crown chakra, our hair, our ears, are all antennas of communication with God and the Spiritual realm. Yes the Divine spark is within us, but our 'antennas' enhance our connection to the higher dimensions. Why would we cover them then, especially when praying or in a place of worship? Religious scribes say it's a gesture of piety which has been culturally and traditionally enforced over the ages.

I don't think this means that if you wear a hat or head covering you are blocking *all* connection, but perhaps it makes a difference.

I know of some hoodoo energy practitioners that advise to cover your head to protect yourself psychically and energetically, indicating that this is a very powerful connection point.

Another instance, is the concept of Reincarnation, and thus the Law of cause and effect. This concept disappeared from Church teachings by way of the council of Constantinople in the year 553. Therefore, taking away opportunities of people taking responsibilities for their lives, gaining independence and security for themselves. If people had understood they were not at the mercy of their fate, or a mysterious judgmental God, they could have understood and overcome a great many life circumstances by gaining insight and changing their ways. The Christian Church suppressed knowledge about this spiritual law of our own, very real, powers of co-creation and being masters of our fate.

Spiritual advancement means we have to turn within, always. There is no guru or any other leader that can facilitate the change we want. We all have our natural gifts within us, our own Divinity, we just have to rediscover them.

The Laws of the Universe

Remember that we are fully responsible for all of our actions, words, thoughts, beliefs, and how we treat others. Even though it's easier to blame someone else, or an energy, or an etheric Being meting out punishment. We can of course receive miracles, divine interventions and aid in our lives, but the state of the world is a direct result of the actions, thoughts, emotions, and beliefs of centuries of humankind.

But if we understand the energy at work in the Universe and how we're completely connected to it and a part of it, we don't have to stay in our current world state. We just need to start to work mindfully in harmony with that energy.

Much has been written on the Cosmic Laws or Laws of the Universe. It's been written about in modern times and also for the past 5000 years in ancient Egypt, Greece and India. A modern-ish study of some of these ancient teachings came out as a book called **The Kybalion** in 1908. Which is a study of the ancient *Hermetica* containing the *Hermetic Philosophy*. Google the words in italics if you're interested in further reading on the topic.

As I wrote this portion of this book, Archangel Metatron came in to assist. He's an Archangel currently very concerned with the trajectory of humankind on Earth. He shares that working in harmony with the energy will require a total re-organizing of our belief systems; societal, personal, interpersonal and familial. Humans deviated from the energy of the Universe over a great length of time but do have the power to correct course and change things for the better.

Through the natural laws below, everything can exist in perfect harmony. There is no judgment or governance with working with these laws, no punishment or reward. No one is taking score. They're simply energetic laws that are impersonal, operating automatically. Consider first how you can apply these laws personally, not worrying about how others do or don't work with these laws. They're in no particular order, all are equal in importance, and all foster harmony in those who practice them.

Law of Divine Oneness
This states that everything and everyone is connected. Everything that we do has a ripple effect and impacts the collective. Every word, thought, emotion and action are intertwined. As we've discussed with the Divine spark, as the energy of God is within us, we are also co-creators, creating all the time consciously and unconsciously. Your thoughts and the dominant emotions of your life become your reality.
This law works fluidly with the next Law of Vibration as well.

How to apply it in your life:
Use willful and mindful application of the power of your thoughts and emotions and focus only on the things you want in your life. Worry and fretting keeps the energy stuck with the problem. You still need to take relevant action but your attitude and feelings have a large impact.

Law of Vibration
This states that the whole universe is a vibration and that everything within it is constantly moving and vibrating, that everything is energy. And like energy attracts the same like energy. This has been referred to as the Law of Attraction. Therefore, whatever you put out into the universe through your thoughts, words and actions

(your energy and persona that you emanate), is what will exactly come back to you. You are like a magnet that attracts people, ideas, circumstances and resources that are in harmony with your dominant thoughts and emotions. Dominant thoughts, not fleeting little thoughts. It's the repetitive thoughts with very strong emotions behind it that we need to be mindful of.

How to apply it in your life:
Match the energy of what you desire and you attract it into your life. Or another way to look at it is, learn how to let go of what you don't want, so you don't keep attracting things you don't like.

Law of Correspondence
This states there is harmony, agreement and correspondence between all the realms. This means that our outer world is a reflection of our inner world and that our current reality mirrors what's going on inside of us. Our conscious and unconscious dominant thought patterns create circumstances in our lives which can help or hinder us. And some of these thought patterns, negative or positive, can be passed down genealogically from our ancestors and family. We can consciously break these thought patterns by changing our perspective.

How to apply it in your life:
By changing how you look at things, the things you look at will change. Changing your perspective.

Law of Duality
This states that everything in the universe has an opposite. There are two equal opposite choices or potential outcomes in any situation. Two sides of the same stick, two extremes of the same thing; hot and cold, light and dark, positive and negative. It teaches that we can

experience both sides of the same coin to fully appreciate them and then we can make better choices based on this wisdom.

How to apply it in your life:
Aim to balance in the middle of the two extremes. At complete balance with everything. It means accepting that a negative experience can help propel you in the opposite direction. You can do this by always perceiving the good in life, even when things seem not so good.

Law of Cause and Effect
Also known as 'what you sow you shall reap'. Every cause has its effect, every effect has its cause. It's also known as the Law of Karma or Newton's third law in the world of psychics. The effect may not always be instantaneous but what you put into the world will eventually come back to you. Even if it's in another lifetime.

How to apply it in your life:
Being very aware and mindful of your words and actions and level of compassion to others.

Law of Rhythm
This states that everything in the universe is moving in a perfect rhythm and everything flows. Moving in a measured motion, like a pendulum. We see this in the cycles of the moon, the tides of the ocean, our own relationships and lives.

How to apply it in your life:
When you feel the natural ebb and flow in your life, try to not let the ebbs cause fear or panic, just breathe through it, perhaps retreat for a little while, and know that the flow will rise again. This means being very strong in your thoughts to not be brought down by what's

happening in your life. You don't hide from it, but your reaction is measured and calm. Over time, the ebbs have less impact because your reaction is more resilient.

Law of Gender

This refers to the two main types of energy in the universe. Feminine and masculine, or yin and yang. Everything that exists has both masculine and feminine elements. They are two complimentary energies which give rise to new creation. In humans, masculine energy is often action and logic oriented, while feminine energy is more intuitive and compassionate.

This law is not related to biological gender. It's about the energies that we all have existing within us.

How to apply it in your life:
Keep a balance of both types of energies within you, as they need to co-exist with each other, so that you feel complete and can live consciously and fully.

Law of Love

Which is love yourself and all others, and all creation.

How to apply it in your life:
Treat others as you would like them to treat you.

Law of Non-Interference

There are two parts to this Law. One, we humans should not interfere with any other humans' path or choices without the other persons' permission. (Aside from life threatening situations) As sometimes people go through things for their soul challenges and lessons and we cannot control anyone else's life other than our own. This also applies to give energy healing or infiltrate their personal energy without their express permission.

Secondly, our Spiritual team can never interfere with our free will. They can save us from dangerous and potentially fatal situations if it's not our time yet, but without us asking for help, they stand by wait patiently, but will not take action unless we ask.

How to apply it in your life:

It's a reminder of your own sovereign power of yourself. No one else can control you and you cannot control anyone else. You can offer help to people, but it's up to them to take you up on it. And also, remember to call in and ask your Spiritual team for the help you need!

As you've read, many of these laws overlap in the complete mastery and self-control over your thoughts, words, emotions and actions, and realizing your own self responsibility in co-creating your life.

The Cosmos

This is our Universe, with our galaxies, planets, dimensions, realms, etheric energies.

There are many reaches and corners of our Universe that we're not aware of yet, where other conscious beings dwell, so my Guides tell me. Souls that also fell long ago and chose to stay in higher dimensions or other planets. Earth as we know it in 2023 is in the lowest dimension, it's one of the most challenging incarnations available and billions of Souls are undergoing life cycles here with the aim of Soul evolution.

Dimensions

A dimension is a frequency band. When you vibrate predominantly at a particular frequency, you reside in that dimension. We humans have parts of ourselves in all the dimensions, we're multi-dimensional. A part of our Soul could already be in a higher dimension.

Physics says we inhabit a space of three dimensions- height, width and depth. And the fourth, which is time. But beyond our Earth reality, our 4D world, there are multiple dimensions, frequencies in the Universal Energy Field. Earthbound Spirits reside in a different, but very close frequency to us. They really are stuck in a place where there is no other life so as I've mentioned, it's for everyone's benefit to move them along for their Soul growth.

The extensive Spiritual help we have available to us come from and exist, in higher dimensions, higher frequencies than us. They consist of higher vibrations and energy and cannot reside in our 4D world for a long length of time. This is why our Higher Self is always connected to the higher dimensions communicating with a whole realm who most of us cannot see. Our communication with this Spiritual team is always clearer when we raise our own vibration and keep our energy clear. They can step down theirs a little to reach us, but not very much. The energy simply doesn't allow it.

There are a lot of resources about the dimensions you can research further. For the purpose of this book, I'm keeping it brief so we can focus on ourselves to navigate this lifetime and hopefully stop the cycles of reincarnation. The infinite vastness of everything is complex and we don't need to understand it all in order to progress individually.

Parallel Universes

My Guides tell me yes, they do exist. *"There is infinite vastness. Just as there are infinite possibilities, there are infinite realities. This is not something that should concern you there on this Earth, nor should it preoccupy your thoughts and efforts."* We are just a tiny faction of our complex Universe and they tell me we cannot hope to understand everything while in a human incarnation. It's more likely to gain this knowledge in the Spiritual realm in Soul form.

The Leylines

These are an energetic grid of the planet Earth, a set moving horizontally and a set moving vertically that provide a highway for Divine energy to flow around the planet. The lines are conduits of energy that course through the Earth, like veins and arteries from her beating heart. The lines have become very clogged and broken down in some places after centuries of humans building, fighting wars, desecrating and disrespecting the land as well as performing atrocious acts against other human beings. All this has an impact on the land beneath.

The leylines, through their grid, also connect high energy and high vibrational sacred sites and wonders of the world. Usually in those places are high energy vortexes with a great deal of natural power. An energy vortex acts like a hub for energy and can bring feelings of peace, clarity, self-reflection, healing, and deepen spiritual practice of prayer and meditation.

Examples of some of these strong energy vortexes are various spots in Sedona, Arizona, the Pyramids of Giza in Egypt, Macchu Picchu in Peru, Stonehedge in the UK, Uluru Rock in Australia, and many others.

But it doesn't have to be a sacred site to have a high energy portal. They can also exist in your corner park, in homes or other places.

And as we live in a world of duality, there can also be lower energy, negative portals. These can occur in homes, in buildings, on the street, anywhere. Caused by many different reasons, but usually from a large change of energy, chaos, a rift from Earth's energy, or some enhanced energy stuck within the veil that is so strong it's affecting our 3D world. What's important is to close these negative portals. This can be done through someone offering space clearings such as myself or another practitioner. And you can also learn to do it yourself with the help of your Spiritual team.

I've experienced both types of portals in different places I've lived. I had a wonderful high energy portal in my home in Dubai, it was in one empty spot of the living room, it was amazing energy and I encouraged the Angels to use it and my home as an even bigger haven of light, of positive energy, to bring more of it into the world. I don't know how it got there but I was very grateful for being guided to rent that home!

And in another place in Canada, before I moved in, I was painting the apartment and after several hours in the empty space I was exhausted, tired, drained, could barely keep my eyes open. Something was definitely up as I was getting enough rest and there was no other issue. I called in a friend to check into the space for me (sometimes two intuitives are better than one! Especially when one is more emotionally vested in an answer) and yes, there was one negative portal in the actual apartment and a few more in the building itself so with the help of my Spiritual team we closed them all and I could feel the difference the next day when I came back to paint.

Sacred Geometry

Sacred geometry reveals that everything is connected. As there is a great deal of sacred geometry in the natural world that correlates with our own cell and body structures.

For example, the Fibonacci Spiral is found in a snails' shell, a pine cone, and a pineapple as well as the cochlea of a human ear, DNA spiral, and human umbilical cord.

Geometric patterns are found from the sub-atomic level to the galactic scale. They can be found in humans, plants, minerals, and everything within creation. It encompasses basic geometric shapes (circle, square, triangle), re-occurring patterns, and numbers as ratios and fractals (a never ending pattern). It creates balance within its formation. It indicates everything is connected and there are no coincidences, just Divine symmetry.

There are numerous ancient places of worship built thousands of years ago that follow sacred geometry in their architecture and art-work. Because using shapes and ratios based on specific numbers was believed to invoke the cosmic forces those numbers symbolized, and this power was used to invoke Deities, ward off evil, and bring prosperity. It was considered a window into the mind of God, the belief that God created the universe according to a geometric plan. Divine order in perceived chaos.

Here are a few examples of sacred geometric shapes;

The Sacred Spiral

The Spiral is one of the most frequent shapes in nature, animals, humans, things related to life and growth. The meaning of the spiral is The Spiral of Life, where nothing is stagnant and unchanging, life is always growing, evolving and moving forward, energy is in constant flux.

You could wear this symbol as a pendant over your heart chakra, placing an energetic vibration of its qualities on your heart as an intention to continue to grow and give yourself permission to let go of past heartache and move forward. Wearing this symbol over your thyroid would be beneficial for physical healing and balancing. Over your throat, for a constant flow of communication, both written and verbal. This shape also forms one of the Reiki healing symbols .

Another way you might see the Spiral utilized today is in a Labyrinth. Walking a Labyrinth, is mindfulness with each step but also weaving a pattern of energy with the Earth. Allowing the energy of Mother Earth and the Elemental beings to work in harmony with your steps to create a positive energy vortex. With a positive vortex, great healing, and clarity of thought can occur, as well as that connection with everything around you. If it's possible, try and walk it barefoot to really connect with the energies. Please note that walking a Labyrinth is a meditative process, it's a particular route to follow with a specific end. It's not a maze which is a puzzle to figure your way out of. This website, https://labyrinthlocator.com/home has a database of labyrinths around the world and there are probably even more.

The Circle
Symbolizing a never-ending union, oneness, completion, a perfect sphere. It can also symbolize the sun and a full moon. This is the reason rings are exchanged in marriages, symbolizing that unending union and together as one. A less positive connotation is a historical symbol of ownership when human slaves had iron rings around their necks or wrists. A symbol of control. Because of the strong power of this symbol, if you do experience a dissolution of a marriage or any

relationship ending, its good energetic practice to sell the wedding rings, bracelets or necklaces that were gifts, or have a jeweler melt them down into something else to release that energetic bond and open your energy to someone new.

The Triangle

Symbolizing the Trinity. in Christianity; the Father, Son and the Holy Spirit, or Charity, Love and Faith. The importance of the trinity, of the three points, of the number three, is a symbol of the connection and unity of the human physical body, the Soul, and God. Mind, Body, Spirit.

The triangle is also used in symbols such as the five or six pointed stars which have their own meanings. Energetically, triangles direct power and intention in the direction which they point or through the middle. At the Casa de Dom Inacio in Brazil, a place of incredible and miraculous healing, the symbol of the triangle is used to direct prayers, requests, and healing energy, as an energetic portal to God and the higher Spiritual realms.

The Square

Symbolizing strength, stability, security, imposing structure on the Earth. The four sides represent a variety of things in our world such as the four seasons, compass directions, the elements, and phases of human physical life (birth, child, adult and death). The number four in numerology also means square, sturdy, solid and balanced.

Many ancient religious buildings were designed using squared-circle geometry, one of the most famous ones is the Hagia Sophia in Istanbul.

Archangel Metatron's Cube

This is a tremendous healing and spiritual tool provided by Archangel Metatron. His cube contains every shape that exists in the universe. By calling upon Archangel Metatron to bring his cube through your aura, chakras and physical body to balance and create harmony, is a quick way to come back to yourself after an immediate stress or trauma. You may need further and deeper healing and balancing with a practitioner later on depending on the situation, but his help is wonderful in the moment when you need to come back to balance and alignment within yourself and the Divine.

Ascended Master Melchizedek .
He's known as an Etheric High Priest with his own order of Light-workers helping the ascension of the planet and humanity right now. He's associated with sacred geometry, colours, and the energy within each piece as movable flows of energy. Remember nothing is static and is constantly fluxing and changing. He helps us with manifesting and shifting energy for a more positive environment. Like with all Spiritual help who abide by the Law of Non-Interference, you must call upon him for his help with shifting a situation or energy.

When to call on Archangel Metatron or Master Melchizedek? Archangel Metatron will assist with a clearing and balancing of your chakras in a quick and efficient way. Master Melchizedek will assist with shifting the energy of a situation or adjusting the energy.

This is just a taste of the incredible sacred symbols surrounding us and within us. I hope it encourages you to research more so you're aware of the meaning and vibration of geometric shapes that you place on your body, in your home, and your vehicle.
This is a good introduction to sacred geometry: Sacred Geometry: Your Personal Guide, by Bernice Cockram

Mandalas

A Mandala, which is Sanskrit for "circle", is a geometric design that first originated in Hindu and Buddhist cultures. The designs represent different aspects of the universe and are used as instruments of meditation, prayer, healing, or teaching.

They're typically produced on paper or cloth, or with chalk, sand, or flowers on stones. They're extraordinary works of art with much symbolic meaning according to whomever creates them. They've been used as a spiritual guidance tool for ages.

Their use and adaptation have become more popular in modern times as a mindful practice to relieve stress. You may have recently encountered an adult colouring book of Mandalas, used to help foster mindfulness in the moment, concentration, or a form of relaxation. Or you may see a wall hanging of one in a yoga studio or for sale in a holistic shop. The idea behind these are to create a sacred space and allow one to gaze upon the mandala as an aid to meditation, focusing the mind.

Significance of Numbers

Do you often glance at the clock and the time always seems to be 11:11 or 3:33 or 4:44? Or do the total amounts on your store receipts show these synchronized numbers as well? You may see it on car licenses plates, or a friend may send a text at 5:55. When these types of numbers keep repeatedly entering your space, it usually means take notice! The Spiritual world is trying to send you a message or letting you know a message is coming in, so take some time to connect and meditate. Or allow for some silence and stillness in your day.

Each number has a specific meaning, for instance some derivative of 3 is a message from the Ascended Masters, 4 is an Angel number, 5 signifies change is coming, 8 is abundance. You can google the spiritual meaning of numbers, and a book I've also used is: Angels Numbers 101, by Doreen Virtue.

Nature's Apothecary

Nature is our great healer, provider, nurturer and apothecary. We are as intrinsically connected to nature as we are to our own energetic bodies. The same Divine Spark that is within each and every one of us, is within each blade of grass, tree, rock, body of water, flower. Within the wind, the sun, the earth, the moon. Within all weather systems and Elementals. Therefore, we are connected at our deepest level with the bounty of nature. From the dawn of time, humans have been surviving and thriving based on what Earth provided, the crops, the ability to clothe, build shelters and receive warmth from fire. Modern times, while blessing us with wonderful technologies, have disconnected us from this cycle and rhythm of connection. It doesn't mean we need to shun all technologies, it just means we have the power to bring more balance into our lives by reconnecting with nature.

The easiest way to do this is to spend regular time outdoors, even only 15-20 minutes if its not the season for outdoor activities. In my sessions with clients, the Angels often recommend at least 20 minutes a day outside; biking, walking, sitting, just being outside. The wind acts like as a giant washcloth cleansing your auric energy. And walking or any physical activity outside is very grounding. Swimming in salt bodies of water do an even deeper cleanse on auric debris. I lived for a time in Costa Rica and the surfers I met had some of the clearest auras I'd ever seen. They spent mornings and late afternoons in the ocean every single day.

We may not all have the luxury of that much time to spend outside, but a little bit per day does make a difference. I myself need to get outside regularly to refresh and rejuvenate myself. Even when I have to drag myself out in the dreary gray skies of winter, I always feel better when I return.

Nature is also a great conductor of messages and signs from the Universe. Any animal or insect that crosses your path can be a deeper message, the unsullied air around you also allows a clearer channel for your own guides to get their messages through.

Everyone wants a view when buying a home. For the beauty sure, but it's also a wonderful subtle healer as you gaze upon water, a mountain, greenery. I have a beautiful big maple tree outside my window that I just like to look at while I write, it inspires me and also allows me to empty my mind to allow the wisdom to come in.

In fact, trees communicate with one another through their root systems, their branches, their leaves, the acorns or food they produce. Entire forests communicate with one another in order to allow enough room to grow, flourish and multiply. I enjoyed this book about this topic: Hidden Life of Trees, by Peter Wohlleben

Only human intervention interferes with this balance. But if we bring back the ancient practices of communing with nature and her cycles, giving gratitude to the bounty provided and not abusing or harming, we can start to re-balance what is off right now. Pan, one of the Deities of the natural wild world advises that this too requires a whole new way of thinking and being, in order to adapt to modern times and yet not ignore the natural world and its effects on us and our well-being. He says we can still have our modes of transport, our infrastructures, our modern conveniences, but to create and build more mindfully with a symbiotic relationship with the natural world, we can all flourish.

The Seasons

This of course varies according to the different parts of the world, but each season has a purpose. The winter, when the trees, many animals and insects hibernate, resting for a time. Spring is a time of new life, rebirth and milder temperatures, where nature starts to produce again after a season of rest. Summer when abundance flourishes with the sun, weather and lighter energy everyone feels and enjoys. And Autumn, a time to harvest and give thanks for the bounty of the Spring and Summer, preparing for the break to come. For the places that are closer to the equator and thus the sun, having little seasonal transition, (except for the rain, nourishing the earth and their crops and vegetation. Cleansing the land each year.) they are blessed with almost constant edible abundance. and with the beauty of modern times, have the ability to send these agricultural products worldwide when other parts of the world may be in winter with less fresh produce available.

Organic Food

Of course naturally grown fruits, vegetables, nuts, seeds, legumes, and grains provide more nutrients than genetically modified or those bathed in chemicals. But at the same time, organic food is just as good as the farmer who cultivates it. How they treat the land, offering thanks and moving in coordination with the cycles of nature? Where do their seeds come from? Also the farmer's attitude, is it loving, genuine and honest? It all makes a difference in the output.

If one non-organic farm sprays chemical fertilizers on a windy day, the wind can easily blow the same chemicals on an organic farm next door. Not to mention all the chem trails contributing to the environmental pollution coming down onto the crops. These days, the label 'organic' on something does not necessarily mean it's actually of a much higher vibration than other 'non-organic' foods. Please use discernment in the food you buy and eat. If you're blessed to be near a farmer's market or locally grown produce, maybe check them out. I find these items are more flavourful as they're harvested when ripe instead of allowing the time needed for transport and harvesting earlier. You could even grow your own food, and then you have full control. That's not something I've tried just yet and I do depend on the grocery store in the winter, but I'm very grateful for all the local produce available to me during the summer months. I certainly appreciate the effort involved in growing crops and like to support local as much as I can.

In any case, anything grown from the earth is still healthier to eat than packaged or processed foods with additives.

Healing remedies from Nature

Remember the Divine spark is in every single plant. And many plants offer great healing benefits to us. In numerous ancient cultures, these were the basis of their healing balms and tinctures for centuries. That knowledge unfortunately deteriorated when just a few hundred years ago, those who knew how to heal with herbs and plants were regarding with suspicion and fear and persecuted for their knowledge. These days, modern medicine rules and anything natural is considered 'alternative'. I'm not negating modern medical advancements, but many pharmaceuticals today originated from a plant or bush that naturally provided an element of the healing.

One example is the bark from a yew tree. A drug widely used in treatment of breast cancer is derived from the yew tree. When I lived in Thailand, dengue fever was very common, with no modern cure. You just had to 'get through it'. But I witnessed the locals treat dengue with the leaves from a papaya tree (brewing them into a beverage) resulting in much faster recovery. Chamomile tea is calming, Ephedra gives energy, Peppermint helps with digestion, there are so many herbs and remedies and I encourage you to read and research further if this resonates with you.

Moon Phases

The phases of the moon offer more or less optimal times to perform ceremonies and rituals. Such as releasing old habits with the full moon and cleansing crystals with the full moon. Some people may sleep less solidly near a full moon or a woman's menses will start at the same time.

A new moon is a time to start new things, start afresh. Some may feel really affected by the moon and like to retreat with a waning moon and feel more energetic and outgoing during a waxing moon. Not everyone is very sensitive to moon phases and we can't blame all our bad moods on the moon, but like with all of nature, we are intrinsically connected to the moon too.

Orbs

These refer to the light filled circular shapes that sometimes appear in photos. They could represent as a variety of colours and are energies of light Beings caught on digital camera. They might be Guardian Angels, Archangels, Fairies, Spirit Guides, or even just passed Souls come to visit from their realm. There's no set procedure to capture these Beings through the camera, they just appear sometimes. This is a photo I took in a very high vibrational place in Brazil. The white orbs are Spirits and the very bright orb is a Guardian Angel.

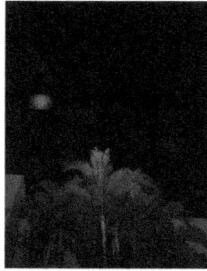

Orbs in Brazil

Extra Terrestrials, Alien Life Forms

Extra-terrestrials, other species, alien life forms. Whatever label you prefer, yes, these beings exist in the Universe. Species other than the humans and animals on Earth that we're familiar with. They are usually (not always) of a higher vibration and more advanced spiritually and technologically and originating from other planets. Their energy is quite different to humans, less concerned and constrained by the physical aspect of bodies and reality on Earth. What this means is that they are very aware of their spiritual natures and the abilities they're capable of. There are aliens of a higher vibration than us as well as those of a darker energy. So, as in everything, discernment when in communication with them is important. Many alien Souls, Souls from other planets, have also incarnated on Earth right now for the great life school it provides. I have a few friends whose Souls originated from other planets than Earth. They never really felt like they belong and are super sensitive in all ways.

There is an Intergalactic Council that is directly involved with Earth and its inhabitants. Their role is to help humanity ascend out of the low vibration and density we're currently in. There are selected high vibrational light Beings who sit on the council, Archangel Michael is one constant on the council as a consultant and bridge with God, while the others are often Ascended Masters and very powerful Beings. You can connect with the council as a whole or to Archangel Michael, to petition how you'd like to help Earth on a global scale, whether for the environment, animals, children, or fellow humans.

(I use the term 'alien' just to define the difference in our physicality. We still all come from one Source.)

The Energy of our Homes, Offices, Cities

Feng Shui

This is an ancient Chinese practice of arranging objects and space in an environment to achieve harmony and balance, in a way that will bring peace and prosperity. It's been applied to the design of towns and homes over thousands of years in the East and becoming slightly more common in the West. Feng means 'wind' and Shui means 'water', both elements which are very fluid.

Feng Shui is concerned with the flow of energy (Chi), the life force and vibration that everything is made of. It's a method to balance the yin and yang energy of a space, improving the flow of energy so that there's more positive energy rather than negative but always a balance. For your home, following Feng Shui principles, by arranging furniture, decorations, and colours can improve the flow of energy. The ancient belief is that arranging these things to create positive energy flow ensures good health, improves interpersonal relationships and brings prosperity. For your office space, it can ensure focused concentration, intuitive ideas and efficient and inspired work.

> Please Note: It's very good practice to keep the toilet lid down in your bathroom at home. A bathroom is one of the key energy centres of a home and having an open toilet is the biggest drain of positive energy in the home.

Why is it important to know all this?

It's beneficial to be aware of what surrounds us in our daily life, and the realm beyond what we can see and touch in our regular routine. Knowing where we come from, what our goal is, what support we have, and how interconnected we all are can help us co-create a life of fulfillment, peace, happiness and purpose. I hope this also incites in you a passion for taking responsibility of your vibration and what you're projecting out into the Universe.

And now on to Part Two to learn who, and what, can help us navigate through the energy and our lives.

PART TWO

The Tools to Navigate Our Path

5

Spiritual Help Available To Us

As you now know, human life on Earth is our school and our Souls are here to learn lessons, make amends, or fulfill a purpose. Since we forget everything we're supposed to do and experience upon birth, we have a multitude of Spiritual Beings available to help us with the demands and challenges of our physical world.

These Beings, who come from, and work on behalf of God, are working overtime to communicate with us. We just need to allow the messages in, and recognize them. Their job is to urge, nudge, encourage, advise, support, and guide us on our life's path. In addition to reminding us, and connecting us, with our Divine essence to live a life of positivity, health, abundance, and personal power, our highest potential. They're available to every single human on this planet. We can easily ignore them for our entire lives but that's like hiring employees to help you run your business (your life in this case), and then telling them to stay home, you'll run it all yourself.

We can call upon them during good times, and during our darkest times. They'll come and go as we need them. If your Soul agreed to a challenging experience, they can't change it, but they can help you through it. They never intervene if it's part of your path, but they do offer warnings and possible gentler alternatives.

The more we ask and call them in for help, the stronger their presence and you'll start to recognize their energy and words. They never interfere with free will, so it's important to ask for help, and then it's also your choice whether you follow the guidance or not. It's still your life, and you, and only you, have complete responsibility for your life.

If you do ignore it, you may get repeated guidance over the years, gentle, never pushy, little signs. They're very patient and are not offended if you ignore them. They may just step back farther away from you if you do.

Usually, the energies surrounding us in our physical world are strong and speak the loudest, while the Highest Self and Spiritual Beings are quiet, sure, loving and precise. So, it's important to spend some time each day, if not in meditation, in silence, in contemplation, in connection with our Higher Self.

There is no limit to what you can ask for and add at the end, *"if this is for my highest good"*, because sometimes something even better is in the works for you that you can't imagine, but your Spiritual team is aware of. Of course, this doesn't mean you can just sit at home asking and waiting for guidance to drop in your lap, you still need to take action, get out there, making decisions and living your life. But you can do so with a Spiritual support team behind you.

It would be remiss not to mention that there are also Spiritual Beings around us who are not of the highest light. I don't mention it to bring in fear, but only to ensure you use your discernment in who you are connecting with and allowing into your energy.

I suggest adding the phrase *"of the Highest Light"* after calling in a specifically named Being. As there are lower energy Beings who are pretending to be some of the more well-known ones and are not helpful at all.

If still in doubt, ask who they are three times, they must tell the truth by the third. Or, you can call in Archangel Michael of the Highest Light first to protect you during communication and also check with him that this Being is really who they say they are. But when you're new to this, I'd suggest to first start with connecting and communicating with your Guardian Angel and/or personal Dragon.

Keeping your physical, spiritual, emotional and mental energy fields as clear as possible helps with receiving clear messages as you don't want any interference or anyone else's energy mixing up the signals.

All of these Beings are available for anyone and everyone to call on for help with the highest intention. They are not limited by religion, race, or culture.

Angels

The word Angel means Messenger from God. They have never incarnated as humans but have been eternally alive as direct reports from God. While some religions depict Angels in their texts and artwork, they are non-denominational and available to all. They may represent as male or female, but really, they're an energy and appear as a gender according to human belief systems. There is no limit to what Angels can help with. Even if you've asked and think, "oh nothing's happened, they're not helping." Rest assured they're working behind the scenes getting everything in place for your highest good.

It does require patience on our part as Angels don't follow calendars or clocks, what comes to you is always according to Divine timing. Angels are very patient. If they've been sending us messages and guidance that we haven't picked up on, they will continue to gently and softly repeat it until we recognize and understand it. Sometimes it takes years for us to notice and take action.

As I mentioned, it does help if we also take great care with our energy and vibration. Angels can help as much as our vibration allows. If we are mired in a very low vibration and thought forms and belief systems, the Angels can surround us and help us as much as our own energy allows them in. The Angels will come when called with the highest intention. For instance, they don't come to help you get revenge on someone, or help to commit a criminal act.

Types of Angels

Guardian Angels

We ALL have our own Guardian Angel, who is closest in energy to us. We all have at least one, and sometimes more come in according to what's going on in our lives. You may feel their presence if you ask them to come closer. They're with us from birth to death and are also aware of our Soul challenges and agreements that we've agreed to in this lifetime. They know more about you than you know yourself! They're your spiritual protector, your companion constantly helping. They protect you from harm that would derail you from your Soul path, unless you ignore the warnings and go ahead with ill-advised action. They also help to bring in synchronicities (there are no coincidences).

They never, ever, leave us. But for some, perhaps with debilitating addictions or life circumstances, who are so out of touch with their inner knowing, they're pushed far back into the aura so its hard to hear the guidance without consciously calling them in closer. Likewise, if you tell them, don't help me! They'll step back but they'll still never leave you.

There is no great skill required to talk to them, they're aware of your thoughts so all you have to do is have a mental communication with them. And then sit quietly or be in a quiet situation in order to hear the answer. Or ask for physical signs for answers. I'll explain further at the end of this chapter.

Earth Angels

These are Angels who descend to our dimension in a non-threatening form, usually in emergency situations, to protect and rescue us. For instance, a client of mine told me of her experience when her car broke down in an unsafe area, she was starting to panic, when a man walked around a corner to her and her car "with the gentlest, kindest, bluest eyes" and was able to do something to the engine to get it going again so she could leave the area and get to a mechanic for a full repair. As she turned to thank him, he had just disappeared. She couldn't figure out where he went without her seeing him walking away. This is an example of an Earth Angel, coming in your time of need and leaving instantly after.

Now, not all people who come around the corner out of the blue may be Earth Angels so please remember to still use your discernment.

Angels of Everything

There is nothing in the Universe that is not overseen by Angels. No blade of grass, tree, flower, insect, animal, or home and building.

Even for things you wouldn't think they could help with. I've asked for help with electronics, plumbing, during air and road travel, even for help with green traffic lights and parking spaces. I just recently asked the Angels to help me at Home Depot. Before I entered, I asked them to guide me to the best staff member who could help me with that I needed. And they sure did, he was amazing.

There are a lot of unemployed Angels just waiting around. Call on them!
They can be with many simultaneously so don't worry that you might be calling them from someone who needs them more.

Archangels

These are the overseers of the Angelic Realm who are dealing with humanity, usually with a specific responsibility they specialize in. I've listed only a few below but there are many more. You can find many resources and oracle card decks with Archangels either online or in holistic shops.

Archangel Michael

He's considered to be the leader of the Archangels and oversees the lightworker's life purpose. He is the best protector Archangel! If we ask, he helps with our confidence and courage and clears away negativity. You can call upon him whenever you feel afraid or vulnerable. He will instantly come to your side, ensuring your safety, both physically and emotionally.

You can call upon him in this way or use your own words:

"Archangel Michael of the Highest Light, please come to me now. I need your help!" And then describe the situation with which you need assistance.

He's also wonderful in clearing your energy and the energy of your home. You can say:

"Archangel Michael of the Highest Light, I call upon you now to please clear my energy/home/airport/office/vehicle/etc of all negative energy and cut all cords from me that are not for my highest good. Thank you."

Archangel Chamuel

This Archangel helps with all types of relationships in our lives; romantic, friends, colleagues, family. You can call upon him to work with you to build strong foundations for your relationships so that they're long lasting, meaningful, and healthy. However, the other person or people always have free will and can decide to stay or go in a relationship, but Chamuel can help with a harmonious parting as well as a harmonious joining.

You can call upon him in this way or use your own words:

"Archangel Chamuel of the Highest Light, please help me with this relationship (describe the issue) Thank you."

Archangel Gabriel

Archangel Gabriel is known for appearing to the Virgin Mary telling her of the impending birth of her son Jesus, and for dictating The Koran to the Prophet Mohammad. And thus became known as 'the messenger' angel. And Gabriel does indeed help messengers such as writers, teachers, journalists, singers, actors, anyone involved in communication in some way. You can also call upon Gabriel to help you overcome fear and procrastination in delivering your message. Gabriel also helps people with child conception, rearing, or adoption.

You can call upon him in this way or use your own words:

"Archangel Gabriel of the Highest Light, I ask for your help with (describe the project). Please open my creative channels so that I may be truly inspired. And please help me to sustain the energy and motivation to follow through on this inspiration. Thank you."

Archangel Raphael

Raphael is a powerful healer for physical bodies, for both humans and animals. He also helps healers and potential healers by guiding them to the right education with enough time and money to study if needed, and helps them establish their healing practice as well as provides guidance during sessions with patients/clients. You can invoke him to heal on behalf of someone else if that person has given permission for spiritual treatment, as he can't interfere with free will. However, if the person refuses, Raphael will still go to them (if you ask) and surround them with a comforting energy which may reduce anxiety in the ailing person.

You can call upon him in this way or use your own words:

"Archangel Raphael of the Highest Light, I call upon you now, I need healing for (describe the situation). Thank you."

Seraphim, Thrones, Dominions

These Angelic Beings have far less to do with humans and are not available to call upon as easily as the Angels I've already discussed. They sit closer to the God frequency and take on a more universal role than only human lives and Earth.

The Seraphim are heralds of God's messages to the Universe.

The Thrones are concerned with the timelines and planetary placements.

The Dominions oversee the Archangels and other Angels.

Dragons

Dragons are powerful etheric Beings from the same dimensions as Angels. They also come from God, just like the Angels. The main difference between the two is that Dragons did come from their own planet originally, were incorporated on Earth for awhile, and then withdrew during the times of hunt and persecution by humans. The ancient legends and lore of Dragons have some truth to them, but keep in mind that humans have written those legends and stories, intentionally creating the Dragons as villains for the most part. They were given the opportunity to leave permanently from humankind but they elected to stay in the nearby dimension, ready to help when we became ready to respect and call upon them once again. They are also blessed with the ability to delve deeper and into darker material than Angels so they are invaluable for their clearing of negative energies.

Dragons, like Angels, go to those who call upon them with the highest intention. They are extremely powerful and should be respected and shown gratitude for their assistance.

Types of Dragons

There are a multitude of Dragons to call upon by name to help with a particular aspect or you can call upon a group of Dragons as a whole for help, without naming them.

Some examples are;

Personal Dragon

We all have the opportunity to have a personal Dragon that we can call in to us. Some people have them with them already, and some need to call them in. They're like our Guardian Angel, with advice, guidance, support, and protection. Connecting and communicating with your personal Dragon and your Guardian Angel is like having two permanent assistants entirely focused on you and helping only you.

Elemental Dragons;

Fire Dragons

You can ask them to clear and transmute with their fire; your own energy, a room, your home, hospitals, earth leylines, and more.

Air Dragons

You can ask them for a soft breeze on a hot day, or blowing rain clouds to or from a place.

Water Dragons

You can ask them for safe passage while on a boat or swimming.

Earth Dragons

You can ask them for help with growing crops or gardens.

Please always thank them immediately after you ask.

Travel Dragons

You can ask them for safe and timely journeys. For instance, on a road trip, you can ask the Travel Dragons and Travel Angels to carry you and your vehicle (and any passengers) safely to and from your destination. With air travel, you can ask them to help your suitcase arrive safe and intact with you at your destination, and then on the airplane, first ask the fire dragons to clear the energy after everyone boarded and then ask them to carry the plane and all passengers safely to the destination.

Arthur Victorious, the Protector Dragon
You can ask him for protection around you, your vehicle, your family, your home, your pets.

Spinnicus, the Healing Dragon
He can assist with all types of healing and oversees the golden healing Dragons who focus on the Meridian energy lines of the body as well as other healing Dragons who assist with specific ailments. As the Dragons say, illness is about flow of energy. Usually something has manifested because its caused by a blockage of some sort so it needs to be removed, dissolved, shrunk, in order to have flow restored. The natural state of the human body is constant movement, flow and regeneration. However, if the illness is part of a Soul lesson or challenge you agreed to, the Dragons cannot eradicate it but they can assist with lessening the symptoms.

What is a Dragomancer?
You feel a special affinity with the Dragons and their realm. Quite probably you've had many past lives working with Dragons and their kin without personal gain in mind. A Dragomancer has been blessed with a spark of Dragon energy in their core, usually just above the heart. A place I call the Dragon Chakra. This was a spark that your Soul accepted and absorbed in a past incarnation from a Dragon themselves. Perhaps in thanks or gratitude for your service and cooperation, or to prepare you for a future role and incarnation working with the Dragons. Reading about the Dragons here and

feeling the most excitement in this part than any of the other Beings, is likely an indication you have a path to work with Dragons in this lifetime.

If you're not a Dragomancer, you can of course still invoke your personal Dragon and any other Dragon for help. You can also activate your Dragon Chakra by tapping on it and offering to work with the Dragons of the Highest Light and inviting their energy in.

Currently the Dragons are coming in to assist with our personal growth and cleansing of the Earth. You can read more about Dragons in my book, Introduction to Dragons.

Ascended Masters

These are Souls who have usually had an incarnation or many incarnations on Earth and have reached an enlightened status and are no longer in the wheel of reincarnation and have been given the option to help humanity and the Universe in etheric form. This is considered a huge honour, and with it is given great power and responsibility to the Universe.

Some well-known Masters are Jesus and Buddha. They have typically been affiliated with religions but with that dogma aside, these are Beings who are greatly helping humanity at this time. Jesus and his Christ Consciousness, which is a spark within us and we can call in as a light to fill us completely, helping us emanate peace, love and compassion.

Buddha can be called upon by those who need help with stilling their mind through meditation, or just being still and silent. He helps those who need focus and a single-minded determination on a task ahead.

There are many Ascended Masters, and if you'd like to read more about them, I found these two books quite informative; Archangels and Ascended Masters, by Doreen Virtue and Divine Masters Ancient Wisdom, by Kyle Gray

Deities

These ancient Beings are the gods and goddesses from various cultures, legends and traditions. They're still available to be called on for help in our lives.
I've given two examples below and their messages channeled for this book. However, there are numerous more you can find from other resources.

Krishna (Hindu)

"I am a light being. I do not have magical powers other than the power and knowledge, the wisdom, to understand energy and the Laws of the Universe, and how to use it. Something humanity could also learn and master at their current dimension. I was created well before any humans walked the planets and embody the emotion of love. That is the true essence of the benign Universe. It is a testament to the humans who kept my story, and my counterparts, alive over the centuries to still exist today. Consider me like an angel in that myself, and other Deities in various beliefs are messengers of God and have a great interest in humanity and their doings. We are all light in different forms of matter. Like with any spiritual guidance, some feel more affinity for me, and some don't. Usually there is a past life connection that resonates with a particular light being which can influence that resonation today. It is not that complicated or complex. You may call upon a specific light being or call upon 'my highest guidance available to me today'. We come to your vibration and requests if it is for your highest good and the highest good involved. Sometimes humans think they know best but they can be very limiting in their beliefs and we can orchestrate something even better in your potentiality."

Brigid (Celtic)

"I represent strength, inner strength and warrior spirit. Often, I am depicted as the ultimate cycle of a female's life - maiden, mother and crone. A full completeness all at once. Many women today feel they are incomplete at certain points of their life. But both men and women are born complete and whole. You have the strength, determination, resourcefulness, wisdom and self respect from birth. A beautiful balance of the masculine and feminine sides of you. It is the human condition that you often forget this and are easily impressionable to your surroundings and teachings when a young age. I can help you forge ahead when you are un-certain and need a guiding light on the way. I can also heed you to wait in place to gain a different perspective on a situation before moving forward. But I am all about momentum, the flux and flow of life, of the Universe and ever changing energy."

Unicorns

Unicorns are beautiful etheric Beings who work with us through our third eye chakra and crown chakras. They are of fey lineage so work closely with fairies and the nature Elementals. Their purpose now is of a far greater reach to help humanity and the planet as a whole. They especially love to do their planetary service work on full moon nights, and you can call upon them in meditation or visualization to travel with them across the planet pouring the purest white light onto people, places, buildings, animals, wherever you'd like to raise the vibration to something purer and lighter. (You may need to visit a few times depending on the energy.) You can also call upon your personal Unicorn to connect with you and ask to be shown your future potential in this lifetime.

They contain the purest of Divine energy in their fields.
The Unicorns are coming forward now to help us reach our highest potential in this lifetime. They are of a very high vibration and work with those acting in integrity with pure intent.

Ancestors

These are individuals who have had a human incarnation and are related to you by blood. You may know some of them from this lifetime, while others lived before your birth and you never met them. However, they are very aware of you and your parents, siblings, aunts, uncles, cousins, children. As I've mentioned previously, as you heal yourself and your karma, you are healing the ancestral lineage behind you. They take a vested interest in your life and while not quite a Spirit Guide (they do not have the same wisdom), they guide you nonetheless. Their guidance is usually oriented toward healing grievances you have with your family, and re-patterning karmic habits in order to release them so you can achieve freedom for yourself.

Spirit Guides

These are individual to you, and assigned based on your life chart and what you need at the time. They have often previously incarnated as a human, and so they understand the human condition very well. The only difference is we chose to come down and incarnate in a physical body and they are having a non-physical experience. Often, they're beings you've had a previous incarnation with and have made an agreement when both in Soul form, that one of you would stay beyond the veil and guide you through this lifetime. They're usually with you for a specific focus or to help you with something going on in your life at the present moment. For instance, a spirit guide may be a monk you shared a past life with to keep you aligned with meditation and spiritual practice in this lifetime. They could have been a lover or spouse. And they fluctuate according to what's going on in your life. If you're writing a book, moving to a new country, starting a new career, or having a child, you can call in your 'writing guides', 'parenting guides', or 'highest guidance possible to help me with this chapter of my life.'

For one to become a Spirit Guide, it takes a lot of training in the Spiritual realms and they always have an Angel overseeing their work.

Technically an Ancestor can become a Spirit Guide after extensive training and if their Soul has reached an appropriate level of evolution.

Animal Spirit Guides

Totem Animal

This is who you are, characteristically. Some ancient traditions link it to your birth date, a little like an astrological sun sign. But you can also sit in meditation or Shamanic ceremony and ask your Totem Animal to come forward.

Power Animal

You can call in a Power Animal to imbue you with their spiritual energy and characteristics when you're facing a particular challenge or for a large part of your life. For instance, if you'd like the qualities of an Eagle, soaring above any problems by taking a higher perspective on issues, you can connect with the Eagle in meditation and ask them to imbue you with their qualities bringing it into your own energy.

Spirit Animal

These are Animal Spirit Guides who appear when we need their support, strength, guidance and inspiration. When an animal or a symbol of that animal shows up to you in an unusual way or repeatedly (at least 3 times in a short period of time) it's most definitely trying to convey a message from the Spirit world to you. For instance, if you go for a walk and see three cardinal birds in that same walk, then I would suggest looking up the meaning of the Cardinal. Or a coyote crosses your path in the middle of the city, or some other unusual circumstance where you see an animal out of place, is a strong sign to tune into that animal and its characteristics on what your message may be. It doesn't even have to be a physical sighting of the animal. Spirit Animals can reach us through symbolic representation. For instance, that would be when you see a beautiful painted mural of a whale on a wall or on the side of a truck, then turn on the TV and a show about whales is on, and then maybe you overhear people talking about a whale watching trip. This would be three literal sightings and message from the Whales. Which you can then look up what is the message from the Whales.

I like to use this book, Animal Spirit Guides, by Dr. Steven Farmer to learn about Totem, Power and Spirit Animal messages and characteristics. Or, you can also google 'what is the spiritual meaning of a coyote' or whatever animal that has crossed your path.

Another option is to sit quietly and tune into the animal, (visualize them in your mind's eye sitting in front of you calmly), connecting with them through your heart and let them know you've seen their notification, and ask what is their message for you. You may receive it as an image in your mind, hear something, know something, or feel it physically. We all receive messages from the Spirit world in our own way.

Elemental Beings

There are also Elemental Beings that exist in nature but vibrate at a different frequency so that we can't usually see them with naked sight. Most of us have probably read about them in books from childhood or seen them in movies. Some may be skeptical about their existence outside of fairy tales. But these Beings do indeed exist in our natural world and their purpose is to serve and protect the mineral, plant and animal kingdoms in nature. Some children and animals see them and interact with them, as well as psychically open people. These little etheric Beings are guardians of our natural world, working with other etheric Beings like Angels and Dragons to protect.

The following are very introductory ways to work with the Elementals, there are many more resources focusing specifically on these wonderful Beings.

Earth Elementals

These are the Gnomes, Goblins, Elves, Fairies who are guardians of each mineral, tree, bush, flower and plant in nature. Their natural home is outside in nature. You can work with the Earth Elementals when planting gardens and crops, asking for their cooperation and help with the plants growth and producing fruit/flowers/vegetables. For those concerned with insect infestation, for example, slugs on lettuce..instead of trying to eradicate them (they are Divine beings as well), you can always plant a few lettuce heads in one corner and ask the earth Elementals to guide the slugs to those specific lettuce heads for their consumption only and to leave the rest alone.

Fire Elementals

These are the fire spirits, the Salamanders. They're in the large fires and bonfires, but also existing within each candle flame. When a fire rages out of control, they're indicating how easy it is for this to happen and is also a warning to humans. With the other Elementals, they help the animals get to safety during these dangerous fires. Fire is a powerful energy, bringing a higher vibration to the area it burns, as well as allowing that light to emanate outwards. I like to thank the Fire Elemental in each candle before I blow it out as they're just doing their own thing dancing around, steadily burning before we put them out, so I like to give them respect for their work.

Air Elementals

These are the Sylphs, the lightest of elemental spirits and can sometimes be seen as wispy cloud formations. They are in the wind, flowing around us, reminding us of the impermanence of things in life. You can ask the Air Elementals for a breeze on a hot day, or for protection of your home during a storm with very strong winds.

Water Elementals

These are the Undines who protect our water and marine life and try to heal the pollution that humans have created in our bodies of water, through energetic purification of the waters. But there is only so much cleansing they can do. Humans do the damage and must deal with the consequences but the Water Elementals will protect the marine life and their habitat as much as they can.

Nature is her own great healer, but she does need time to do so.

When to ask for Help?

There really is no limit. Any time of day or night, from any place. Nothing is too big or too small to ask for help. Health, abundance, career, love, peace, your garden, a project, an idea, home, family member, in relationships, healing an animal, travel, parking, traffic, safety in driving, shopping, in negotiations, with decisions big or small, time management, studies, conflicts. The list is endless. Just be clear with what you're asking for help with and from whom. Intention is everything in calling on Spiritual help. Look at this support as a council of very wise Beings who know your past, present and best possible future outcomes. They're familiar with your Soul self and you've likely crossed paths when in Soul form. Remember when asking, you can end your request with *"for my highest good"* to ensure you do not limit yourself. Sometimes we ask for things we think we want, but they know something even better is available.

I have guided meditations available on my YouTube channel to meet your Guardian Angel, Personal Dragon, and your current Spiritual team to help you get started. Later on, as you become more adept at connection, you'll start to recognize new guides who've come in. And of course, you can call in on any Being I've mentioned above without having to 'meet' them first in a guided meditation.

How to Ask?

Intention is everything so the medium of asking is less important. You can ask out loud, ask in your head, ask in your journal, write a letter, or ask during meditation. Just use your words to ask for help and say thank you immediately after asking. It shows faith that you know your pleas have been heard and will be answered. Gratitude energy attracts more of the same blessings, we don't say thank you for their egos.

The specific words you use are less important because higher light Beings always respond to your true feelings and desires. So, it's not *how* you ask, it's only *that* you ask. If you're unsure of what the exact outcome you want is, briefly explain the situation and ask for help *"for my highest good"'* and they will know exactly what you need.

Try not to let fear or begging into your request, as that clouds up the energy with a lower one. And once asked, LET IT GO. That's a big part of it, asking, then having faith and trust you've been heard and will be helped.

For instance, if you're in a restaurant and you order salad from the server, you order it once, secure in the knowledge that the server will bring you your salad as soon as it's ready. You don't keep asking the same question each time the server passes by. It's a similar premise in asking your Spiritual team.

To ensure you're connecting with only the highest light Beings, you can say this prayer before you tune in:

Prayer of Protection:

I now call upon Archangel Michael of the Highest Light. Please set aside my ego for the duration of this session and realign me with my Higher Self and the Divine. Help me be a clear intuitive channel for messages and guidance, under grace in a perfect way. If any spirits enter this session who are not for my highest and greatest good, please remove them for their own progress and prosperity.

Another option:

I now command everything in, near, around, above or below me that is not of light, to go back to where you came from. So be it.

I know sometimes there's fear in connecting with the intangible and unknown, I experienced it myself! But we must always remember,

1) We have the absolute power and authority of our bodies and energies so we can command and forbid what we don't want. With confidence.

2) Our home is our sacred space and we have the right to command lower Beings out of it. Sometimes they're sticky ones, and in that case I call in Archangel Michael and/or a Dragon for help.

3) Faith that Light always prevails over Dark. Call in the big guns; God, Archangels, Angels, Dragons, Ascended Masters. Not so much the Ancestors or Spirit Guides, their role is different. If I wake from a frightening dream, the first thing I do to calm my racing heartbeat is call in Archangel Michael of the Highest Light to clear the energy of the dream and visualize him doing so, and then I recite the Lord's Prayer or whatever prayer comes to mind until I calm down.

How are the Answers given?

The guidance and answers can come in so many forms as we all receive information and learn things in our own unique way. If you hear it in your head, it's subtle, loving and gentle. You may mistake it for your own thought. Or you may hear a one word answer, or a yes or a no. You may hear a conversation nearby, hear a certain song on the radio, or you may notice physical signs like repetitive number groups, feathers, coins, animals, birds. An idea may drop into your head in the shower, or while washing dishes. Stay aware and alert to what's around you and coming into your energy field.

Usually noticing a physical sign three times or more in a short period of time is a message from the Spiritual realm. And sometimes an ending (being fired for instance) or an upset which moves you into a different direction is also the workings from your Spiritual team with long term benefits coming.

We're in this life 50/50. Meaning we ask for the Spiritual help who immediately come to our aid, but we also have to do the work, the action, the effort on our part.

They can only help and advise so much as we are here on a learning experience. They can't make all the decisions for us, but they help our lives stay on, or get back to, our right paths, helping us through the good times and the hardships, trying to help us experience as gentle an existence as we can, in accordance with our Soul agreements.

Fear abounds on our planet these days. But we must always remember that the light, the good, always wins, it just takes persistence. Don't let the chaotic noise in our world destroy the joy and faith in your heart. Know that you are always guided, protected, supported, and loved! Know that your Highest Self, acting through your own intuition, will keep you out of harms way and help you manifest the goals you want to achieve. Know that in life, everything is possible!

6

Using Your Sixth Sense

You know that everything is energy, we're energy, we exude energy, everything around us is energy, and our interactions with others and ourselves is energy. Now what? What do we do with this information in order to improve our daily lives? How do we work with the energy?

Calling on your Spiritual team is one support system, you can also ask for guidance and help from a psychic, intuitive, and energy practitioner, and you can also learn to develop your sixth sense, your higher sensory perception of the energy around you.

Using your Psychic Senses

We all have these senses to some degree. We most certainly ALL have intuition which is constantly giving us signals and feelings to guide us on our path. We also have our psychic senses that may lay dormant in some, and others have a barrage of overwhelming information coming to them. Its not a matter of comparison as we're all on our own path, but we can practice and develop and enhance these senses. We can reawaken them and fine tune them like a muscle, the same way a professional athlete does in their sport. Some people's senses are more prevalent because of their individual soul path and the skills are perhaps nurtured and encouraged from childhood. While for some children, any competence shown may be dismissed and shamed into shutting down as 'not normal'. These children may reawaken their gifts later in life, or forever leave them dormant. Usually a person has a natural flair or dominance in one of the abilities but can develop the other abilities with practice.

It doesn't necessarily mean you'd have to become a professional psychic, but working with these subtle energies and gifts will help you navigate life choices from a place of innate wisdom, making better decisions.

For instance, reading a vibe/energy of a person and feeling whether its a wise choice to go into a relationship or business partnership with them. Sensing the subtle energies around you and understanding them. It's not about becoming a fortune teller or doing party tricks, it's becoming a more sensory Being.

Using your psychic senses is like tuning into the energy that surrounds you, others, and your environment. You are like a tuning knob on a radio, tuning your vibration to either connect with a spiritual Being and their vibration, or tuning into someone's energy or the energy of a place to read the room or situation.

As we discussed in Chapter 1, we hold all of our thoughts, feelings, experiences, belief systems, desires, regrets, our whole essence of our being is emanating from us all the time, within our auras and energetic bodies. So by developing our higher sensory perception, this is the energy we are tuning into. And you can learn the ability to control it, so you're not bombarded with information whenever you step out your door.

For any Marvel fan readers, you may remember in the 2016 movie Doctor Strange, when Dr. Strange is asking The Ancient One how does he get from here to there (harness energy with his hands), The Ancient Ones asks "How did you get to reattach severed nerves and put a human spine back together bone by bone?" To which Dr. Strange replies, "Study and practice. Years of it."

I never forgot those lines because it struck such a cord within me as being very true. I reawakened my psychic gifts later in life and the more practice and work I did, the better and sharper I got.

Having a Mentor or a Teacher

I have had several during my journey and I am eternally grateful to them for their teachings and guidance. They all had their own unique gifts and provided me with a well-rounded education and training. If developing your abilities is resonating with you, then I suggest start with a course, or a workshop, or a program, with practitioners who you resonate with. Starting to use your senses is the first step to bring out your natural psychic gifts. You may find one trusted teacher or mentor who could consistently guide you over time, or you may want to experience different teachers and check in with an intuitive once in a while. There are so many options and paths available to learn further so you have to do what's right for you. This kind of learning isn't done overnight. Feel free to email me at natome44@gmail.com for recommendations if you're interested in this path .

To really make full use of your senses, its helpful to keep your own energy and aura crystal clear so you can be a clear channel and have clarity on the messages received. This means at the same time, doing your own inner work, healing and releasing trauma and burdensome energies. As you do so, you'll find your senses come in even sharper.

I also do not recommend doing any psychic or energy work while under the influence of alcohol or drugs. While they may lower inhibitions, they also open up your energy to lower vibrational Beings and negative energies who could enter your fields and cause havoc at the time and later on.

Types of Psychic Senses

Clairvoyance
This is 'clear seeing', and indicates you have the ability to see Beings, energies and visions. Either with the naked eye or in the mind's eye.

Clairaudience
This is 'clear hearing'. Being able to hear etheric voices and messages, either from within the head or as external sounds.

Clairsentience
This is 'clear feeling'. Also known as an empath. This is the ability to tune into the atmosphere in a room or to experience other people's emotions or physical distress as though it were happening to you.

Claircognizance
This is 'clear knowing'. When you just know things without being told and receive fully formed ideas and information about a person or situation. Often this sense comes hand in hand with Clairsentience.

Clairgustance

This is 'clearly taste'. You perceive a flavour that is not physically present. For instance, a Psychic Medium may be communicating with your passed grandmother and taste lemons in their mouth. Your grandmother's baking specialty may have been lemon meringue pie. It's one way that information is transmitted from Souls who've passed, with a reference from their earthly life as not all Souls are very talkative to tell a Medium pertinent things.

Clairolience

This is 'smell clearly'. It's similar to Clairgustance. You might get a waft of perfume that makes you think of your grandmother or smell pipe tobacco from your grandfather.

Synesthesia

This is when senses cross over each other to give a greater awareness of what's going on. You hear music and see colours in your mind, or taste food and feel their shape as round, sharp, or square. Or you simply experience all the above psychic senses all at the same time.

Telepathy

This is the ability to transmit words, emotions, or images to someone else's mind without speaking out loud or having any physical interaction. This can be done with humans and animals. Trees can also communicate this way.

This is the method used in animal communication. This video, The incredible story of how the leopard Diablo became Spirit - Anna Breytenbach of communication with a black leopard in Africa is a great example of this.

Mediumship

This is cooperative communication between a living human individual (the Medium) and the Soul of a passed person who has experienced physical death.

Mental Mediumship

The communication occurs through the Mediums' own consciousness through their clair senses. The Medium calls in the Soul and then relays what they feel, sense, see, or hear to the client. Usually a person would ask a Medium to be the 'in-between communicator' with a passed loved one or friend for closure, or just to have reassurance that they're okay. Other Souls could also come through who the client only knew peripherally. This is because word spreads in the Spirit realm, and Souls get excited that this is a chance to communicate with the living and be understood. However, Souls still have their free will and it's up to them whether they come when called. While others don't even need to be called, they'll just come when they know their relative or friend has booked a Mediumship session.

Trance Mediumship

This is a form of mental mediumship in which the medium blends with the Soul in a subdued consciousness. From light control where the medium is still present, to stronger Spirit control where they directly speak through the mediums voice, and to the most advanced Spirit control when the medium is no longer present in their own personality and the Spirit speaks, acts and advises through full control of the Medium's mind and body. This is also called Unconscious mediumship, where the medium is 'asleep' during the spirit's visit and remembers nothing afterwards.

Personally, I would not do this type as I wouldn't want to give up control of my body and mind to anyone.

Physical Mediumship

This is when the Soul present manipulates energies to produce manifestations like loud raps or noises, voices, objects or apparitions. This is witnessed by everyone present and was all the rage in seances in the 1800's when they were extremely popular.

It takes a lot of energy for a Soul to physical manipulate in our world, but some do have the ability, even outside of a Seance or Mediumship session.

Channeling

This is when the channel (the live human individual) is receiving a flow of information from an etheric Being. Channeling can come through the channel via speaking, healing, automatic writing, artwork, music, really any creative output. The channeler can do this intentionally and with purpose or it can come through spontaneously without control by the channeler. However it comes through the channel, the information comes via one or all of the psychic senses and how much the channel allows in. Our ego self does not give up control easily! We can all channel to an extent as the act of channeling is receiving Divine wisdom and guidance from God, an etheric Being or your own Higher Self. Remember, the universe is nothing but a constant sending and receiving of energy vibrations and frequencies.

There are some people who are currently channeling higher wisdom from a specific or a variety of light beings to share with the rest of humanity. Please note that not all channelers who share their messages are getting their wisdom from THE highest light Beings. Again, it's best to use discernment in who you listen to. Your own inner wisdom and Higher Self guidance is usually the best barometer for you.

Other ways to receive Guidance and Messages

Meditation

'Monkey Mind', you may have heard the term before. It's when your mind keeps jumping all over the place to different topics rarely settling on one for more than a few seconds. So no decisions are made, or clarity achieved. Breathwork, meditation, walks in nature, affirmations, journaling, these are all ways you can calm your mind full of chattering and screeching monkeys. I say from experience, it takes practice! One of the first times I meditated was for 10 minutes (I had a book I was following) and I lasted about 4 seconds before other thoughts came barreling in, none of them related to each other, and I found that by the end of that meditation session I had composed my to do list for that day and ruminated on an argument I had earlier. The monkeys had taken over!

It took a lot of perseverance and practice to get better at letting my thoughts go for a period of time. I moved to guided meditations because that helped me focus on the visualizations and I got great results that way. Eventually as I progressed, I dropped the guided ones and did my own meditation which is really sitting in silence and focusing. Sometimes my mind still wanders but I let it go and then come back to my focus.

It's really what meditation is. Focusing your mind to let the thoughts flow out and you're left with a tranquil mind with no actual thoughts.

Why not try it yourself now? Close your eyes, focusing on your breath flow for a moment, then with the next inhale, count 1, and with the exhale, count 2, and with the next inhale count 3, and the exhale, count 4, and so on until you reach 17. Then, open your eyes.

Were you able to completely be in the moment, just breathing and counting with no other thought? It's okay if not, keep practicing and you'll get there. It's allowing for that stillness and silence in our mind to allow serenity and messages to come in.

Many people tell me they can't meditate or it causes them even more anxiety to try, and in that case don't force it. Walking in silence in nature, or driving in silence, can also be forms of meditation. It's the moments without distraction.

How often? Daily.

Prayer is asking of the Divine, Meditation is listening to the answer, Ceremonies are setting an intention and Rituals are action being taken.

I was once in meditation where I felt this incredible connection for a moment. It was like a wave of immense peace, love, calm, surety. I was enveloped with this incredible feeling that everything is absolutely perfect, all is good, I am good and it will forever be good. It was like every worry, insecurity, fear, limitation, concern and care evaporated, as if I had never felt those things ever. It was a moment of pure, conscious bliss. It felt like all the energy of Jesus, Buddha, Mother Mary, every single Angel, God, was being poured into me. Amazing! And it only lasted a few minutes. Afterwards, I tried to analyze what did I do before this particular meditation to bring that on? Was it the breathwork, what did I eat, or not eat, what had I been doing or thinking before? I still don't know what brought it on but wow, if I could live within that conscious bliss at all times, nothing at all would EVER bother me and I would just float serenely through life. I came to the conclusion that it was a blessing to be shown that state of being and attainable with continued self-work.

Dreaming

Is as natural a process as breathing. Only overuse of alcohol and drugs could prevent dreaming. Those who say they don't dream, are just not remembering their dreams.

What do dreams mean though? The interpretation and understanding of dreams is a form of divination on what your subconscious, your Higher Self is telling you. On some occasions, what your Spiritual team, or passed loved ones are conveying to you during sleep.

These messages you receive while sleeping can foretell your future, reveal your past that needs clearing, warn you of danger, offer creative inspiration, assist in releasing obstacles in your life. Dreams can be a doorway to interdimensional travel and communication.

There is an abundance of resources on dream symbology and while it's helpful to consult them, also remember that the symbols you receive will have a personal meaning to you as well. So use these symbol dictionaries as a method to help you find your own interpretations. For instance, you may dream of diamonds, and one dictionary will say it represents your hidden facets shining, or not shining. Another may say it's a warning that a great temptation will come. Or it could represent diamonds your mother wore and indicate some unresolved feelings with her. Or simply mean a desire for more abundance, depending on the context of the diamonds in the dream. Sometimes the symbol is a metaphor for something. Only the dreamer can really know the true meaning of a dream.

Lucid dreaming

This is when you're sleeping and dreaming and then suddenly become conscious that you are dreaming. You become aware that you're dreaming during the actual dream. These dreams tend to seem as real and vivid as waking, conscious reality. This is something you can practice and become more proficient at over time. The value of lucid dreaming is that it's a way to connect more deeply with your Soul, allowing you to address trauma or personal limitations, as well as remembering your true essence. I myself have not done this, but you can research more about it online and the Institute of Noetic Sciences offers workshops on this.

Dreamcatchers

These items are not tools to receive guidance but I was guided to include their role in this section. They originated with the Indigenous cultures in North America and have become more common and widespread today. The original ones are handmade objects made of willow and sinew, fashioned into a loop (to represent the earth's spherical shape) with a web woven on the inside of the loop with beads or charms woven in. They usually have feathers hanging down.

These were used to hang above cradles to protect babies from illness or other harm. The bad dreams would be caught in the web to stay until the sun came up and burned them away and the feathers would be transporting good dreams onto the baby or adult (nowadays) sleeping below.

Astral Travel

There are two forms of astral travel when we explore the multi-dimensional universe. One is when you direct your consciousness to 'travel' in mindful meditation, and the other is when your energetic body, an aspect of your Soul, travels. This aspect remains corded to your physical body from the solar plexus chakra. Sometimes if you wake up suddenly in the middle of the night, this is your energetic self coming back in for a landing.

Most of us astral travel while we sleep, upon the decision of our Higher Self to learn, help or progress. You can also request the same before falling asleep. For instance you can say, *"Higher Self, I would like to astrally travel tonight to the temples of higher learning in the Spiritual realm so that I may gain knowledge that I remember in my conscious life to help me on my life path"*. The final decision would still remain with your Higher Self as they have the higher perspective of what is best for you.
You can also ask Archangel Michael of the Highest Light to protect you astrally and physically while you sleep.

Dowsing

Dowsing has traditionally been the act of finding a hidden water source, minerals or crystals deep in the Earth using a tool held by a person. The person using the tool is usually also tapping into their own intuition in finding these items.

A **Pendulum** is another dowsing tool and one more commonly used today. It's usually a crystal, or stone, or wood piece, usually a natural element, hanging from a chain. You hold it at the top and ask the pendulum questions that ask for a yes, no, or maybe answer. The pendulum itself is not magical but is attuned to its owner and the owner must set the intention when using the pendulum to connect it with their Higher Self and the highest Divine wisdom within. If you're in an unprotected space, you can ask Archangel Michael of the Highest Light to protect you while asking the questions of the pendulum so he keeps away all lower Beings who may sully the answers.

However, we are such powerful beings, that sometimes if we're very emotionally tied to the answer (we want a yes for instance as a no would be distressing), we can influence the sway of the pendulum. So it's a good idea to ask before your question, *"May I have unbiased answers now when I ask about xx?"* You should always be relaxed and calm when asking the questions. If you're in an agitated or tense state, you may not receive clear answers. Also asking once is enough, if you keep asking the same question over and over, the answers get muddier.

Please note, if you purchase a pendulum, it should be energetically cleared (Chapter 8). Then you should sit with it in mediation or holding it in your hand as you walk outside so that it becomes charged with your energy. When not in use, keep it in a safe place like its own pouch. If someone else handles your pendulum, you'll want to do the cleansing and charging process again to get it in tune with your energy once more.

Psychic Readings

I like to also call these sessions **Holistic Life Coaching**, because you're asking for guidance from a higher perspective, addressing all aspects of your life; past, present and future.

These are technically external methods of receiving guidance and answers, because you're asking another (human) individual to read the energy. Which is something many intuitives and energy practitioners do as well every once in awhile. A reading can provide confirmation of what you're feeling and thinking, and its helpful to know if you're on the right track.

And often, an objective third party can best advise your possible future outcomes better than yourself no matter how spot on your intuition is. As our strong emotions and what we desire may cloud our intuition.

What is a Psychic?

Someone who sees and/or senses your energy and the energy surrounding you. Seeing into your energy fields of your past, present and potential futures.

What are they actually sensing? The energy within you, around you, your past timelines, other people's energies within yours, animals close to you, present energies or situations you're in, the state of your chakras or auras, your physical imbalances, and current possible future outcomes. I say current possible future outcomes because we all have the power to change our future from different choices that we make. There's a general path for you that a psychic sees that seems inevitable, but can be slightly, or largely, changed if someone, not just you, makes a certain decision.

Some psychics also call in high level Spiritual Beings to assist during a psychic reading. As these Beings are residing in the higher realms and can access higher knowledge and a greater perspective to help identify any blocks and potential next steps.

As with everything, choose a professional psychic that you resonate with, perhaps someone recommended, or ask your Spiritual team to guide you to the right one for you.

Akashic Records

These are the energetic library of information that contain details of your Soul and its journey from all past lives, present incarnation and future possibilities. They contain the entire history of every Soul since Creation and these records connect us to one another (through the collective consciousness). The knowledge of their existence came into the mainstream in the 19th century, but for centuries the Records were the exclusive domain of mystics, saints and scholars. This is no longer the case as humans have been growing and evolving spiritually. We now all have the awareness and ability to access our own Akashic Records.

The Records exist in another higher dimension called the Akasha. There, every thought, idea, and action from the past, present and future is stored forever. It's like a database of what's happening, or will happen in the Universe. The Records tell you what the most likely outcome is going to be based on the trajectory you're already on. But of course, with your free will you can decide to go down a new path and redirect your possible outcomes. With some training, you can access your own Records, and there are also specialized Akashic Record readers who can access them on your behalf and be an impartial message relayer to your questions.

Astrology

This is based on the premise that you are a reflection of what was happening in the Cosmos the moment you took your first breath.

Because of the exact time, date and location of your birth, you take on the essence of that moment and place. However, your astrological sign and charts do not control you. You still have free will on your life path. It simply reveals who you are, based on your entry into this lifetime. I like this analogy...at the time of your birth, visualize a camera hovering over our solar system, using YOU on the Earth as the centre of the photograph. A picture is taken at the precise moment you took your first breath, a picture showing the positions of the Sun, Moon and the planets and how they were arranged around the Earth and you. From your perspective here on Earth, everything from the solar system revolves around you, you stand in the middle, and that is your astrological chart. A living representation of that moment in time and place when you were born in this lifetime on Earth. As you grow and time passes, the planets in your chart continue to move around you, these are called planetary transits. Astrologists use the patterns of the planets, stars, Sun and Moon to forecast earthly and human events.

Numerology

Numerology is the study of numbers and their direct energetic influence on our lives. A numerology reading is based on your birth date and full birth name and can be used to help you find direction and meaning in your life.

While there are many online tools to provide you with your unique numbers, usually a comprehensive reading would be done by a Numerologist to provide a more detailed and accurate reading. They would create your chart by calculating your numbers and their energetic impact. Things like your life path number, your soul urge, expression, and personality numbers and how they work together is what the numerologist interprets for you. This meaning can help you understand yourself better as well as discover insights about your purpose and personality traits and identify your strengths and weaknesses.

Divination Tools

Divination is the intent to seek knowledge of the future and the unknown. These ancient tools have been used in Divination practices for centuries among many different cultures and there are probably even more than what I've listed below. The tools themselves are not magical, although should still be treated with respect, but it's the interpretation by the user's intuition that provides answers. Anyone can use these tools as they usually come with a little guidebook to help you at the start.

Cartomancy (Divination with Cards)

This is the practice of consulting a card deck in order to read someone's (or your own) past, present and potential future. Using card decks as mystical tools have been around since the 15th century. Tarot card decks were one of the first to be used for fortune telling and mysticism, with the more modern Oracle cards of all types, coming onto the market in the last 40 years or so. As I've said, the cards are not magical. The talent lies within the reader of the cards, and as they shuffle while tuning into the energy of the client, or their own energy (if doing a self-reading). It's how the reader interprets the cards for each client that make them portentous.

I myself use Angel Oracle cards during my psychic readings but at this point in my evolution, they're loose guideposts of the message and I find much more of the information and guidance comes through my clair senses and the Angels I call into a reading. But when starting out, the cards were a great source of comfort and support while I built up my confidence. They helped to match what I was seeing, feeling and hearing with my clair senses while I was drawing the cards.

I Ching
Is a system used to predict the future for oneself, and as a book of wisdom through the explanations, which are simple, profound and intuitive. It has been consulted for advice and insight into human nature, the universe, and ethical life for millennia.

Rune Stones
These originate from the ancient Germanic and Nordic tribes of Europe. Today, they consist of 24 letter symbols, the runic alphabet, carved into wood or stone that are cast for readings to provide guidance, advice, and foretelling of that the future may hold. The messages interpreted are largely dependent on the intuition of the person doing the rune reading.

Tasseography
This is a fortune telling method that interprets patterns in tea leaves, coffee grounds, or wine sediments. The reader interprets the symbols in the sediment of the cup you've just drank out of. The interpretation of the leaves, grounds or sediments are embedded within their shape, density, colour and placement, and the intuition of the reader.

NATASHA TOMÈ

7

Holistic Healing Modalities

The premise of Holistic Healing is to heal the Mind-Body-Soul connection. You know that we are more than the body and while we are blessed with the modern medical industry to heal the physical, the Mind-Soul aspect is equally important. History shows that ancient healers coming from cultures in Egypt, China, India, Greece, Rome, the Celts, and all Indigenous cultures from the Americas to the Australian Aborigines were advocates of healing the whole holistic connection Many of these ancient practices supported the need to cure the energetic bodies prior to any permanent physical cure could be achieved. In short, to heal the root cause, a human must be considered in their wholeness - Body, plus Mind and Soul.

Energy healing is just one expansive tool at your disposal, with many modalities and focus areas. Since we're all unique individuals with different lives that shaped us to be the person we are today, what might work for one, may not work for another. Try a method that resonates with you, and ensure the practitioner is operating with integrity and skill.

But remember, for true effectiveness, we need to care for ourselves as a whole package. This includes; energy balancing and clearing, medical treatment (if you need it), the food and drink you ingest, movement of your body, releasing the past, mindfulness of your thoughts, words, actions, and what and who you allow into your energy. True change comes when you combine all the best practices to make a difference.

To help you in your journey of well-being, I've included a list of Ho-listic Healing modalities in this chapter. These are ones that I know of and have tried, or been trained in, but there may be many more available. Energy healing all works in the same way in that it helps to clear energy blockages and brings into your body and energy fields, the Universal Life Force Energy, and activates your own body's innate healing and life force energy to promote balance and optimal flow of all body systems.

Coming from a strong enough place, the body has the mechanism to heal itself through the more subtle energies flowing within the body that contribute to healing.

While many of these practices are considered 'New Age', they're actually quite ancient with roots established thousands of years ago. We're blessed to have this information resurface and become more widespread in order to help us experience the health, abundance, power and joy available to all of us.

I must point out, for some people, Holistic Healing sessions may bring up long repressed and buried trauma and emotions. This is part of your body's innate healing and Higher Self wisdom to bring the things which are heavy and burdensome up and out. It can be part of the process to feel it all before releasing. But it IS the process, it serves no one to keep it all inside imprinted into your cells and energy, we must release them.

Please note, I am NOT recommending you stop any medication or medical care prescribed by your Doctor. Please continue with your Doctor's advice, but know that learning how to work with the energy within you is a complement to medical protocol and contributes to your overall balance and well-being. You are a unique, beautiful, and perfect Holistic Human consisting of many nuances and layers.

Energy flows where intention goes, so some of these modalities are equally effective with distance healing as well as in person. While others are specifically hands-on treatments.

Acupuncture

A part of Traditional Chinese Medicine and involves the insertion of solid, thin needles along the meridian lines of the body. Placement is dependent on the ailment. The point is to correct imbalances in the flow of energy within the body.

Acupressure

This is the same premise as Acupuncture but without the use of needles. The practitioner uses their fingers to apply pressure on specific points of the body depending on the ailment.

Angelic Healing

Invoking Angels to help with healing and balancing can be used alone or in conjunction with another modality such as Reiki, Atlantean Healing, Crystals and more. You can call in Archangel Raphael and the Angels of Healing throughout any healing session.

Aromatherapy

This is when quality plant essential oils are placed on various parts of the body, or diffused into a space. This can help with mental, emotional, spiritual, and physical imbalances.
I have been to Aromatherapy workshops arriving with tension and a headache and leaving three hours later feeling fantastic when all we did was smell a variety of oils!

Atlantean Healing

A modality that was used in the healing temples of Golden Atlantis. During sessions, the Angels from Golden Atlantis are called in to balance the energy field. Atlanteans believed disease was a manifestation of imbalance in the energy field.

Auset Temple Healing

A system based on ancient Egyptian healing methods and alchemy founded by Australian Healer and Psychic Elisabeth Jensen.

Ayurveda

An ancient system of traditional medicine from India that does not exactly involve energy healing, but does view the body and mind as a whole. It's a healthy lifestyle system that emphasizes good health and prevention and treatment of illness through behaviours and practices such as dietary change, meditation, yoga, massage and herbal remedies.

Bach Flower Remedies

These are the dilutions of flowers developed by Edward Bach, an English bacteriologist, pathologist and homeopath in the 1930s. The flowers used impart specific qualities to the remedy. Remedies are usually taken orally and are safe for pets.

Barbara Brennan Healing Science

Barbara Ann Brennan is the author of books; "Hands of Light", "Light Emerging" and "Core Light Healing". She writes about the human energy field and developed an intuitive system of hands-on healing which combines an overall holistic approach involving the spiritual and psychological state of mind.

Bio Magnetic Therapy

This uses a variety of magnets of different sizes and polarities. The magnets work by improving circulation to the damaged cells in the body which speeds up biological processes and enables the body to reduce inflammation.

Bowen Therapy

This is a therapy that involves manipulating fascia, muscles, liga-ments and nerves. It helps release tension and stress in the body and mind. Over a series of sessions, the body's autonomic nervous system responds to the work, allowing the body to restore itself to a healthier state.

Breathwork

Is a conscious adjustment of breathing patterns to release energy as well as induce calm peace.

Chakra Balancing

A regular chakra balancing and clearing should be done as maintenance for optimal health and well-being. Most energy healing practitioners include this as part of the session.

Chromotherapy (Colour Healing)

Colours have their own vibration and energy which harmonize with our own energy systems.

Chromotherapy is a treatment method that uses the visible spectrum of colours through visible light to cure. When the colours, with their unique vibrations, are combined with a light source and applied to the area of the body with the ailment, it's providing the necessary healing energy required by the body for healing.
Light affects both the physical and energetic bodies, and colours generate fields of energy that activate biochemical and hormonal processes in the physical body.

Therapies aside, colour also has a huge impact on our moods, ranging from what we wear, to how we decorate our homes, or even the colour of car we buy. Its very personal as to what colour resonates with a person and often someone's favourite colour can indicate that is the energy lacking in their life so they seek more of it from a sub-conscious level. I encourage you to research further on the various colour meanings but here are a few common ones;

Red   Action, leadership, passion, anger
Pink   Love, affection, compassion
Purple Psychic ability, intuition
White Connection with the Divine, purity, cleanliness, innocence

Craniosacral Therapy

A gentle hands-on technique to examine membranes and movements of the fluids in and around the central nervous system, from head down to the tailbone. The point is to relieve tension in the central nervous system.

Crystal Healing

Crystals have their own vibration and benefits to our energy systems. This involves placing relevant crystals on different chakras or parts of the body to allow the healing qualities of the crystal to impart into the body. This is often combined with another modality.

Crystal Bed Therapy

This specifically comes from the Casa de Dom Inacio in Brazil and is something I use in my healing practice. It's a special kind of chromo-therapy machine, and when the lights and colours are activated through the seven clear quartz crystals, this creates a healing portal for the healing Entities to come in and work on what is needed most. Sometimes going as far back as removing past life and ancestral energy trauma. Each session also heals and balances the chakras.

Dragon Healing

Like Angels, invoking Dragons to assist with healing and balancing can be used alone or in conjunction with other modalities. I often call in the Dragon of Acupuncture when I'm receiving acupuncture to activate the needles with more life force energy. I ask him to 'amp it up'!

Eden Energy Medicine

A modality using tapping, massaging, tracing, swirling, ans connecting specific energy points on the skin and along energy pathways to ensure flow, balance and harmony within your systems.

Emotional Freedom Technique (EFT)

A tapping method using your fingers on the energy meridians in the body, and also incorporating psychotherapy to reach emotional issues that may have caused the energetic disruption.

HeartMath

This is a meditation technique focused on moving from a state of stress to a state of calm. It's done through heart focused breathing to align all your systems to work in coherence.
The HeartMath Institute conducts research on the heart-brain connection if you'd like to learn more.

Homeopathy

Homeopathic medicine are natural remedies derived from plants, mineral, insects, and animals which provides miniscule doses of the ailment to stimulate the natural immunity of the body to cure the ailment.

(When I took a course on acute homeopathic care, I learnt that the AMA (American Medical Association) used to have a predominance of homeopathic practitioners who were pushed out by the influential families of the time who saw the value of their medicines and used them to found the pharmaceutical giants of today for much greater profit.)

Hypnosis or Hypnotherapy

This is a tool used during a therapeutic process to assist you to change certain undesirable conditions and help heal from past traumatic experiences.The process is when a hypnotherapist guides you into a deeply relaxed mental state (somewhat trance-like) with verbal cues or imagery. The intent is to go deeper into the subconscious to help achieve therapeutic goals. Not everyone can be deeply hypnotized, it's how much you're willing to let go of control.

Iridology

This is when practitioners examine a person's iris and compare what they find with iris charts, which divide the iris into zones that correspond to specific parts of the human body. A person's eyes in this case, are windows into the body's state of health.

Jin Shin Jyutsu

Originating in Japan, this modality balances energy by adjusting the flow of energy through the body by focusing on key regulation points of the body energy flow.

Muscle Testing

While not really a modality, its a tool used by many to speak to the body and the Higher Self by viewing how the body physically reacts to a question to determine if it's a yes or no answer. You can google 'muscle testing' to learn more.

Quantum Healing

Is a movement or manipulation of energy to a better state of being. Utilizing our mental, emotional, spiritual and physical aspects in order to transform the energy.

Naturopathy

Not quite an energy healing, but Naturopathic doctors diagnose, prevent, and treat ailments by looking at the holistic person as a whole. Rather than just suppressing symptoms, they work to identify underlying causes of illness and develop personalized treatment plans which usually utilize lifestyle practices such as dietary change, environmental factors, reduced stress, supplements and body movement.

Neuro-Linguistic Programming (NLP)

This is a system of changing someone's thoughts and behaviors to help achieve desired outcomes. Affirmations are a tool of NLP.

Past Life Regression

A method that uses hypnosis to guide you to memories of past lives and incarnations with the aim of releasing negative energetic impacts from those lives affecting your current lifetime.

Pranic Healing

A non-touch modality that corrects imbalances in the energy field of the body by applying frequencies of energy to the relevant areas.

Psychedelic Plant Medicine

Plant based hallucinogens have been used in ceremonies around the world for centuries. In the 1960's in North America, the 'hippie culture' were most known for indulging but also during that time, there was a great deal of scientific research into these plant medicines as potential to treat trauma. The political climate soon put a stop to that but it's currently having a resurgence. There are more clinical studies going on today and also a culture of plant medicine retreats, workshops, and experiences taking place all over the world. Ayahuasca, Psilocybin, and Iboga, are some of the plants on offer and I strongly suggest fully researching the facilitator providing the environment and the source of their plants before taking part. Traditionally, the Shamans would start with thanking and honouring the plant spirit, and cultivate accordingly for the highest healing benefit of all. Along with further ceremony and ritual to keep all safe and of a high vibration.

Some less scrupulous facilitators may add things to the brew to make it 'more trippy' or strong. It doesn't mean you have to travel to South America to take part in something authentic, just do your research and tune in with your Higher Self to assess if it's for your highest good.

Qigong (pronounced chee gong)

Is a combination of moving and breathing exercises which balances the body energy and promotes relaxation and strengthening of the body.

Raynor Massage

This is not like a traditional massage, as it focuses on the muscles, the skeletal system and the subtle energy systems of the body. If the tension in the body is from emotional or stress related reasons, this disrupts the flow of life force energy, and can cause an area of the physical body to become tight, or forced out of position which the practitioner will then use their hands to manipulate the physical part combined with your breathwork to release.

Reflexology (Foot)

This is not just a foot massage. This is where a practitioner presses, pokes, or rubs various points on the foot and toes to reflex body organs for their stimulation and balancing to release blocked energies in the various organs. There are also hand and ear reflexologists.

You can google 'foot reflexology chart' to learn about the organs associated with the parts of the feet.

Reiki

One of the most well known energy healing modalities, Usui Reiki, originated from Japan in the 1920s. The practitioner places their hands gently on various positions of the head and body, transmitting the Universal Life Force Energy through their hands and Reiki symbols into those positions of the receiver. The intention is to unblock energy and restore balancing and healing to the chakras and body.

Tai Chi

A series of body movements and breath to create proper flow and balance of Chi (energy) throughout the body.

Shamanic Healing

An ancient healing art practiced by many Indigenous cultures worldwide. A Shaman, also known as a medicine person, leads the person on their shamanic journey with various natural methods and spiritual help.

Shiatsu

Originating from Japan, the practitioner uses pressure from their thumbs or hands on the meridian lines of the body to ensure flow and unblock stuck energy. A form of Accupressure.

Sound Healing

Healing by sound is possible because our human bodies are not solid. Our bodies are ever moving and ever changing. When there's an illness, it means we've gotten out of tune and our body's vibration has lost its rhythm. There are several different aspects of Sound Healing...

Solfeggio Frequencies

These are specific tones of sound that heal and soothe the body and mind. You may have heard these as background music during a yoga class, guided meditation or other sacred ceremony.

They're tones in sync with the natural rhythms of the universe, which have been used in Sanskrit chants, by Gregorian monks and other ancient spiritual practices. They originated in the 11th century, and came to the forefront in the 1970's when researchers found that the original six tones were mathematically in tune with the universe. The Solfeggio Frequencies are tones vibrating at certain hertz frequencies that resonate with our brainwave hertz and are also associated with the energy within our main chakras. You do not need to listen to these tones with headphones.

The original six Solfeggio Frequencies:

Healing effects on the mind and body:

396 Hz – Liberates Fear and Guilt (Root chakra)

417 Hz – Facilitating change/Undoing patterns (Sacral chakra)

528 Hz – Transformation and Miracles (Repairs DNA) (Solar Plexus chakra)

639 Hz – Connecting/Relationships (Heart chakra)

741 Hz – Expressions/Solution (Throat chakra)

852 Hz – Awakens Intuition (3rd eye chakra)

In the 1970's, researchers applied the same mathematical patterns to uncover three more 'modern' frequencies:

174 Hz - Relieving Pain and Stress
285 Hz - Cellular Repair/Healing Tissue
963 Hz - Divine/Higher Consciousness (Crown Chakra)

If you'd like to learn more about the tones, there are many resources online and if you'd like to listen to them, I often use Meditative Mind's YouTube channel, but I'm sure it's also available on other platforms.

Binaural Beats

These Beats work similarly to the Solfeggio Frequencies except that you must wear headphones while listening to these tones. First discovered in the 19th century, this is how they work; a different tone frequency is sent to the left and right ears through the headphones. When the brain hears the two different frequencies, it interprets one consistent and rhythmic frequency. This frequency is the mathematical difference between the two tones sent to the right and left ears. For example, the right ear receives a 205 Hz tone and the left ear receives a 200 Hz tone. The difference that the brain hears is 5 Hz, which corresponds with the Theta state of our brains, the state of deep relaxation. The brain then follows the 5 Hz tone and produces brainwaves of the same frequency. In this example, producing a state of deep relaxation to match.

The jury is out on which method works better, for many it's a personal preference, and for some, a necessity. For instance, if someone is deaf in one ear, then Binaural Beats won't work as one must hear with both ears with the headphones on. In that case, Solfeggio Frequencies may be more suitable. Try what resonates with you.

The Music We Listen To

There has been research that discovered the effects from a type of music played and the correlating physical effect on the human body. In the 1980's, Dr. Glen Rein tested the impact of different music on human DNA. He exposed DNA in vials to four different kinds of music – Gregorian chants, Sanskrit chants, Classical and Rock. By measuring the rate of UV light absorption (an essential function of healthy DNA), he was able to assess the reaction from each type of music. The chants had the most positive healing reaction by increasing the UV light absorption between 5-9%, the classical music increased it by smaller amounts and the rock music decreased the UV light absorption, harming the DNA. Dr. Rein's research supports the theory that sound frequencies yield major effects on our well-being.

Chanting

When you lift your voice in ritual, you are amplifying your intent and broadcasting it to the universe at a vibrational level. Often as children, we're told not to be so loud, or that we have no talent for singing and at a certain point we can believe it and stop singing, chanting, or even speaking our truth at all. As an adult, we might continue telling ourselves that same story that I can't/shouldn't sing, or I need to stay quiet so I don't bother people. These are old restrictive beliefs that we can send packing immediately. The beauty and strength of the human voice belongs to everyone. You have a voice, and that voice has power.

When chanting, you can choose a Mantra or chant what someone else has written, or chant your own words. Chanting is a healing modality in the sense that it opens and clears your throat chakra. It's also another form of meditation, a way to enter a state that quiets the chatter of the mind and brings you into the present moment. The words are important only as far as they take you to the state where you can be deeply engaged and connected.

What's a Mantra?

These are sacred recitations that have been used in spiritual practices in many cultures for ages. The words may invoke protection, communication with God, peace, purification, they can really cover anything and everything. Either spoken aloud or internally within your mind, a Mantra creates a sense of energetic vibration around your body. Just like sounds from musical tones and instruments, the repetitious chanting of Mantras emits a reverberation of energy and vibration of the thing you're trying to invoke. It's important to chant with awareness and mindfulness of the words you're saying, and if it's in another language, to understand exactly what it means in your language. The words, your intention, and the vibration from your vocal cords, and brainwave patterns while chanting the Mantras are very powerful.

Drumming

A drum is one of the earliest types of sacred instruments and very prevalent in Shamanistic traditions and Indigenous cultures. Holding the drum in one hand and beating it with the other, is a rhythmic form of drumming representing the heartbeat of humans, animals and Mother Earth. Its purpose is to induce a trance-like state in order to access the Spiritual realm.

I experienced a healing session with a Shaman where she beat the drum for 90 minutes while she went into a trance-like state and called in all the healing Spirits to work on healing my energy. With my eyes closed, the sound was hypnotic, rhythmic and relaxing and I fell into a sleep-trance-like state for most of it. It was a very tranquil experience.

Singing Bowls
(also known as Tibetan Singing Bowls and Crystal Singing Bowls)

You may have seen or heard these bowls during yoga classes, at wellness retreats, in holistic stores and centres. In addition to the traditional uses for spiritual ceremonies, they're used today to facilitate Sound Baths, enhance meditation, aid with healing, clear energy, and promote feelings of relaxation.

These bowls may be made of metals, or more recently, crystal quartz sand. For centuries, they've been used in Tibet and surrounding areas in spiritual ceremonies. The ancient ones have been made of metal and when struck with their appropriate mallet, the bowl vibrates and produces a rich deep tone. The vibration and tone produced depends on the size of the bowl, where and how you strike it, and where it sits. They 'sing' when you strike them.

Since the 1990's, crystal singing bowls have been used for Sound Baths. These are healing experiences where there are numerous bowls, that could be all crystal or metal, or a combination of both, and the practitioner strikes and plays them to produce waves of sound for those lying down in the room. The sound vibrations produce a healing, relaxing and meditative experience.

Tibetan Bells (Tingsha)

These are two small cymbals attached by a leather cord. The cymbals range from 2.5-4 inches in diameter and when struck together, produce a clear and high pitched tone that clears the energy around it. They're often used in prayer and rituals by Buddhists. I use mine to clear the energy after each client session, as well as to clear any stagnant energy in parts of my home.

Tuning Forks

These were invented in the 18th century and traditionally used to tune musical instruments as they work by releasing a perfect wave pattern to match the instrument. They cover a range of Hertz frequencies for many uses. The fork consists of a handle and two tines, when hit with a rubber hammer, the tines begin to vibrate and the back and forth vibration of the tines produce disturbances of the surrounding air molecules. These vibrations stimulate chi, the body's energy flow. So striking a tuning fork, then holding it against the area that feels painful or tense on the body can encourage healing.

If you'll remember from Chapter 3, our physical bodies are largely made up of water and water conducts sound, and therefore the body is a wonderful resonator for sound. Sound resonates over four times faster in water. So these vibratory sounds travel through the body to help the energy flow and stimulate the body's natural healing abilities.

Why do we need to know all this?

While these modalities use different techniques and procedures, their common intent is to;

 - unblock and clear stuck energy in the body and its energy fields for optimal flow
- balance the body's physical and energetic systems (mind-body-soul) for optimal health

- release trauma stored in the body and mind
- promote self-awareness as a Holistic Human

Here you have a wide array of choices to help you treat your holistic self and practice self-care. Sometimes it's only one modality needed for a few sessions, and then adding another into the treatment protocol, or sticking with the same one until you improve. It depends on the individual and their condition to know how many sessions are needed.

Of course, not everything stems from emotional and mental imbalances, sometimes a physical injury is just an injury and it needs physical repair. Energy healing can also complement the physiotherapist or other treatment you're on. Any shock to the body, whether tripping, in an accident (but physically unharmed), falling down on the ice (or falling anywhere), the shock reverberates through your energy fields so they could use a balancing after the fact. As well if you have physical surgery, this can leave a tear in the aura, which can cause you to leak energy. It's good practice after you've recuperated from the surgery, to have an energy healing session and specifically tell the practitioner that you'd like them to check for tears and holes in the aura for sealing and healing.

And sometimes the illness is just an illness, maybe you caught a cold or got a flu virus and it's your body talking to you, saying slow down and rest while you recover from this.
Or a disease could be from a Soul agreement or Karmic reason. Then, in addition to the medical treatment, energy healing can help ease symptoms and help in a way that your Higher Self allows. If it's someone's time to pass on, we can't interfere or change that.

8

Practical Tips and Tools

I call a comprehensive approach to our complete well-being; physical, mental, emotional and spiritual - Holistic Hygiene. Like physical hygiene, it's important to take care of it every day in order to bring in the greatest results. This means being mindful of your emotions, mental state, energy (or you can call it your spiritual aspect) and physical feelings.

If you're disconnected from these aspects of yourself it's like communicating with the universe through a heavy blanket around you, muffled and shielded from your full potential in this lifetime, and everything just seems so hard!

In this chapter, I'm providing practical tips and tools to help you incorporate into your own daily routine for optimal balance. These are suggestions and you can of course modify to what resonates with you. Your intention, persistence and dedication are what's important.

Enjoy the new adventures and experiences coming to you!

The Physical Aspect

Nutrition

There's a great deal of information circulating on diet and spiritual awareness and awakening. There are many practices, from Breatharians, Vegans, Ayurvedic Doshas, and more. What I've discovered through my own journey, client sessions and guidance from the Spirit realm, what you eat and the choices you make for your body are very individual and should be true to you, not to a dogma or another's restrictions. Usually eating fresh nutritious food is the highlighting principle, as well as all in moderation. Quality over quantity and avoidance of packaged, pre-made food that has preservatives added. Food from the Earth is normally what the Angels say.

Some may be guided to vegetarianism or veganism while others want animal protein. Choose what feels right for you. If you eat meat and fish, bless it before you eat it, thanking the animal for giving its life for your food. An animal's flesh will hold any fear they experienced in life and at the moment of death so this is something to keep in mind within the energy of the food. This is the appeal of free range and humane practices for where the meat comes from, as well as wild caught fish as opposed to farmed. Much higher energy vibration.

But hey, we're human, sometimes we just want 'comfort' food (I'm not sure who first called it comfort food but what a great gimmick!), pizza, cheesecake, French fries, copious amounts of chocolate (or is that just me?). If a large part of your diet sits in this category, don't beat yourself up about it. Your body will resonate with your thoughts. Your cells, organs and systems will feel it and respond accordingly if you eat a chocolate bar thinking, "oh this is so bad, I'm so bad for eating it, this food is so bad". Instead, advise your body "we're getting this amazing treat that is so tasty and wonderful and we're going to enjoy it so much."

When I first learned Reiki, my teacher taught me to bless my food with the words *"I bless this food with the love of God, may my body only absorb the calories and nutrients I need, and all else pass right through me"*. This gives the food a little added vibration boost.

Of course, we still have to be mindful of our food intake, even blessing a diet consisting of fatty, fried and sugary foods would still have a detrimental effect on our health over time.

Another tip for when eating out, cut the energetic cords from the dish (I use the palm of my hand facing the food and swipe it over the dish, cutting cords.). This is to detach the energy from the one who prepared the meal. The reason for this, is that you just want to be eating the food, not the chef's sadness over a recent breakup for instance!

What the Angels often say is, it's all about moderation. Eat mostly fresh and nutritious foods from the Earth and love your body, in any shape, state or size.

Movement

Try to incorporate some type of body movement each day if you're able. A simple stretch routine, yoga, tai chi, qi gong, a walk in nature, a fitness class, a gym visit, whatever makes the blood start pumping and your circulation system become activated.

There's a great deal of content for free on YouTube of all of the above gentle options. I like to follow Yoga with Kassandra's YouTube channel, but you can also put Tai Chi, Qi Gong or Stretching in the search engine and find more.

Cosmetic and Cleaning products

It's also good practice to be mindful of the products we place on our skin, our largest organ, as well as the household products we use to ensure we're not inhaling harmful chemicals on a regular basis. If you must clean with these products, protect yourself by wearing gloves, or a mask to protect your mouth and nose from inhaling anything toxic.

Grounding

While we are Spiritual Beings first and foremost, we do have a physical body rooted in this reality, so for balance, it's best to be grounded into Earth and also connected to the higher realms. When you're grounded, it's easier to be in the present moment, organize your thoughts and stay in alignment with your goals. When you're ungrounded, you may feel stressed, easily distracted, spacey and unconnected to your body or life.

There are things you can do which will naturally ground you; walking normally or some type of activity outside, walking barefoot on the Earth or sitting with your tailbone on the Earth, physical exercise, eating a heavy meal (particularly of foods like potatoes that have been grown underground).

But I recommend doing this daily, every morning, and repeat as needed throughout the day, this visualization to ground yourself.

Visualization to Ground Yourself

Sit or stand.

Close your eyes.

Visualize tree roots going down from your tailbone (if sitting) and from the bottoms of your feet (if standing) deep into the Earth beneath you, see them going down, down through all the soil, sand, rocks, right to the centre of the Earth and wrap your roots around the crystal pillars in the centre of the Earth.

Visualize your roots being wrapped around a huge pillar of black obsidian crystal. You may also get your own visual of another crystal or something else that your roots wrap around, and that's fine. Once your roots are wrapped, visualize they tug down a little bit, really anchoring you in.

Say thank you to the Earth for her bounty and open your eyes.

The Mental Aspect

As you've read throughout this book, the thoughts you think have a large influence in creating your reality and contributing to your overall well-being. For instance, when you feel overwhelmed or your mind keeps spinning and you can't seem to calm your worries, this is when you take a time out to get yourself calmer and centred. Even if it's just a few minutes to breathe deeply in a bathroom stall at work. Or a walk around the block. Just taking a moment without your phone, interruptions, or anyone else infringing on your space helps stop the downward spiral. It's also a perfect moment to call in your Spiritual team to help you with whatevers going on. The problems don't go away but you can start to handle them from a less tense place.

Mindful in the moment

This the practice of staying in the present moment as much as you can. Not fretting about the past or worrying about the future.

Focusing just on what you're doing this minute, hour, or day. It's not an easy task but if you can achieve it even for only part of your day, then you've already shifted the energy within and around you. Everything benefits this way, whatever task you're doing gets your undivided attention, or you're enjoying a day off and appreciating the sun shining, and you didn't send any worry energy ahead to the future or expend pointless energy on what's already happened in the past.

Of course, you still learn from the past and set goals and plan for the future. Being mindful means you don't worry or feel anxious about either.

It's a conscious decision to stay in the moment and keep your mind focused, remember Monkey Mind from Chapter 6? I spoke about Meditation there, and will repeat again, even 10 minutes a day of meditation will be beneficial for a calmer state of mind.

Affirmations
Affirmations are positive statements that can help you overcome self-sabotaging thoughts and negative thoughts. The science behind it involves the neuroplasticity of your brain. Neuroplasticity is your brain's ability to change or adapt. Which means that your brain can continue developing and changing throughout life, as can your belief systems.

For instance, before attending a job interview, some may say to themselves *"I'm awful at interviews, I don't know how to sell myself well, I probably won't get this job"* but by saying an affirmation such as this before the interview, *"I am confident in my ability to present myself and I am fully qualified for this job"*. It doesn't mean you automatically get the job, but it can help you approach the interview a bit more calmly and answer questions with confidence.

Affirmations are not magical spells that once said, things miraculously appear. That would be nice! But affirmations are able to provide you with a step toward change, by being mindful of how you're thinking and describing yourself.

It's important to use present tense in your affirmations, as you're declaring who you are to the Universe and sending that energy out. Attracting much of the same vibration. You still have to take your action steps but they'll flow better with a positive mindset.

Examples:
"I AM healthy in all ways right now"
"I AM lovable as I am"
"I have the power to make this happen"
"I AM confident"
"I AM intelligent and capable"

As with many things in life, patience and perseverance is required. For some, energy may shift quickly, for others, it may take months or years. Remember, we're all on our unique path, so don't give up, you have nothing to lose by maintaining positive self-talk and self-belief for your lifetime. Make it a permanent change, you'll even attract other positive self-talkers and believers. People who resonate with your energy, your 'soul tribe'.

Content coming in
It's not just our own thoughts affecting the tranquility and balance of our mental state.
We also absorb a lot of information throughout our day. From other

people, radio, TV, the internet, books. All this content carries an energetic vibration that we soak into our physical and energetic bodies. So please be conscious of what you're allowing yourself to soak up.

You don't have to ignore it altogether, but the less time spent on negativity and despair the better. I have felt energetically dirty if I spend too much time scrolling on social media. And sometimes after certain TV shows or documentaries.

Boundaries

The same applies to your valuable time spent with others. If you feel drained, exhausted, burdened, riled up, depressed, after speaking with or being around some individuals, it could be time to set some loving boundaries, placing yourself first. You may have heard the term 'energy vampires', these people may not even consciously realize they're doing it, but sometimes they are very aware of it and leave their meeting with you feeling great after dumping all their stuff on you. When you're in their company and talking with them, they are energetically feeding off your (usually) much higher vibration and draining your mental and emotional energy. So that when you part, you feel exhausted and drained. I'm not saying start ghosting needy, co-dependent friends or family, but please think of your own energy and perhaps limit the time spent, so that you don't come out of the interaction feeling worse than before you started. Your self-care above all else.

My guides recommended I expand on this topic, so here are a few tell-tale signs of an energy vampire:

1. Whatever's going on in their life, it's never their fault. Often in victim mode.
2. Some kind of drama often surrounds them.

3. They like to feel superior to others.
4. Very little time is spent on what's going on in your life when you're together.
5. They use emotional manipulation (guilt, shame, criticize, bully) to take advantage of your helping nature and time spent with them.
6. They're co-dependent in most relationships.

What can you do?

1. Establish boundaries.
This is easy to say I know, but you can do this with baby steps, like saying no sometimes instead of always yes. Put a limit on text exchanges if it's occupying a large part of your time.
2. Adjust your expectations.
You won't be able to change them, but you can limit your response and reaction.
3. Limit time spent together.
Listening unendingly while they vent, is another form of no boundaries. You can try listening to the problem, offer firm advice, (or not, depending on how you feel) and then leave. Ask yourself, are they really after a solution, or do they just want sympathy and to be told they are right? Therefore, making this a repeat occurrence since no solution is ever applied.
4. Cut them out of your life entirely.
You have the freedom to do so, because in the end you are protecting yourself. For some family members, this is not always possible. If that's the case, then remember that spiritually, you chose this family for a reason, try looking at the higher spiritual perspective of why and what lessons have to be learnt by yourself. Their lessons are their path and are out of your control.

And of course, we're not leaving these people out in the cold, but ultimately, its beneficial for them to learn to take responsibility for themselves and use their God-given strength and power to make constructive changes in their lives. Others can help them sure, but the main responsibility and intention lies within. That goes for all of us. We cannot depend on another human being to make us happy. That places too much obligation on the other person, and it can be taken away at any moment. Happiness really is an inside job.

Sometimes your workplace can consist of an environment of many energy vampires. In that case, ask the Angels before each shift to pour a column of white light down into your workspace, wherever you spend most of your time there, and envision it covering you within that pillar of light. You may need to refresh it mid-way through your shift. By bringing in Angel energy every single day, you will undoubtedly raise the vibration, even incrementally, and at the very least, allow yourself to feel less affected.
You can also call in the Fire Dragons of the Highest Light to go in overnight and clear your workspace's entire building of all lower, dark and dense energies. Do this once you're at home, asking them to do this work while you sleep. You can do it every night, or just once, sense how the energy is afterwards.

Everyone has an Opinion
If you find yourself spending a lot of time with negative, judgmental, or gossipy people who really bring your mood down, it's okay to retreat and nurture yourself. That type of talk is very low vibrational and remember that you are the Master of your high vibrational self and energy! The same goes for arguments, you don't have to convince anyone of your beliefs nor justify your actions to anyone. You

don't need anyone else's approval, other than your own.
When we can release these drivers, we free ourselves beyond imagine.

If someone is pressuring and pushing their beliefs onto you that you simply do not resonate with, you can calmly say 'we can agree to disagree' and end the conversation. Releasing the need for anyone having to be right and 'winning'.

You are your own sovereign power and authority, to do and say what feels right for you. Start to tune into your intuition so that you can be discerning with all those who enter your life.

The Emotional Aspect

The Past

There are many facets that make up our emotional state of being. There's our current situation and life experience and also our past. Everything we experienced from the womb, birth, childhood and in adulthood made an impact on our energy, emotionally, mentally, physically and spiritually. This means there may be inner child wounds, rejection and heartache from relationships, abandonment issues, emotionally distant parents. As you've learned, children are like sponges for the first seven years of their lives, even if effects don't show outwardly, little triggers, wounded child energies can be inserted and stay forever. A child may have heard they're stupid or fat (so no one would love them) or not deserving of love because of something they did, bringing these beliefs into adulthood and running an underlying subconscious program with their relationships, choices and self-confidence.

And then as we mature into adulthood, energetic cords develop with other people in our lives, sometimes burdensome cords which don't do us any good and tie us to another self-defeating pattern. And we emanate this amalgamation of our energy into the world.

So to that end, it's very good practice to do the work to release all the burdens, all the 'baggage' from your past. And for some people, release past life imprints as well. This can be done with an energy practitioner or therapist, but you also need to do the work to release. The sessions can get you started and then it's a daily effort to shift your mindset and take action.

Get in touch with me if you'd like more information on how to do this with an energy practitioner. You could also research the more conventional counselors and therapists that are near you or available via Zoom.

In the Moment

Then there's our emotional state in the moment. It's a good idea to check in with yourself emotionally each day, assess how're you feeling, are those emotions your own or did you pick them up from someone else? Since our auras extend outwards a few feet from our body, when we walk amongst many people, we can pick up others emotions and energies. The world around us is an energy soup!

And especially after a strong, traumatic or unfavourable emotional conversation on the phone or in person, you need to cut your cords with that person to stop that negative energetic link which can be draining or keeping that emotion vibrating strongly within you, overshadowing more peaceful, harmonious emotions of your own.

This is especially important for those in counselling and healing positions, it's good practice to incorporate an energetic cleansing routine (tips you'll find later in this chapter) between each client, and at the end of each work day so you don't take on the energetic burdens of others.

The Spiritual Aspect

Intention and visualization are a large part of spiritual practices. It's an energy link from our Soul within our physical shell to the energy we're calling in. Thus you'll find in the forthcoming tips, instructions to always visualize as you say the words either out loud or in your mind.

Cleansing and Clearing

Personal Cleansing and Clearing Methods

1. Visualize white Divine energy pouring over you like a shower. Transmuting all the negativity surrounding you with the light. Let the white light flow all the way from the top of your crown, into your core, down into the ground. You can affirm "I am completely cleared now".
2. Burn White Sage or Palo Santo or use an aura spray.
   Use it over your entire body, front and back, over your head, underneath your feet and armpits, and between your legs to clear out negative energy.
   You can also clear your home and vehicle this way.
3. Fresh air, Sunlight.
   Get outside in nature for a walk or sit outside and ask Mother Nature and the Elementals to cleanse your energy of auric debris.
4. The Violet Flame
   Call upon St Germain and Archangel Zadkiel to place the violet flame around you and visualize yourself in the middle of the flame cleansing your body and aura as if you're on fire. Also direct it into each chakra, cleansing each one of all you're

ready to release.

You can also ask that this be done to your home and vehicle.

5. Vacuuming with Archangel Michael.

   Call upon Archangel Michael of the Highest Light and his vacuum Angels to join you now. Ask them to vacuum all areas of negativity and energy not your own from your aura and body. You can visualize them holding a vacuum over your head, or using a handheld one to vacuum all this murky energy away.

   You can also ask that this be done to your home and vehicle.

6. In the shower

   Ask the Water Elementals to use the water to cleanse you physically and energetically. As the water pours over your head and body, visualize it's also clearing you energetically. Thank the Water Elementals.

7. Sea Salt Baths

   This is one of the best ways for dispersing of negative energy and clearing auric debris. Place 2 cups of natural **Sea Salt** (this is different to Epsom salt, Himalayan salt, table, and kosher salt) into your bathtub. Soak for a minimum of 20 minutes. If you don't have a bathtub, you can take a handful of sea salt in your hand using it as a scrub over your entire body. Then soap and rinse as usual.

Cutting Cords

We form energetic cords all day long, with people we speak with, have strong emotional interactions with, or people we help. The energetic cords connect the two of you, so it's very good practice to cut them off your body at the end of each day so that your own energy is not being drained and you're not bringing the other's persons energy onto you.

Daily

You can do it yourself, stand up and use the edge of your hand as if it were a blade and brush it down (lightly skimming your body) over the front of your chakras, over your head, under your feet, behind you (as much as you can reach), under your armpits. Cords can develop anywhere, not just into chakras. White Sage alone will not remove cords.

You can also call in Archangel Michael of the Highest Light to cut cords from you that are no longer serving you.

Or, you can listen to my meditation: Clearing with Archangel Michael (7min) and visualize as I guide you through Archangel Michael's clearing.

After a Relationship Ending

This applies to any long term relationship, but especially romantic ones. This is so you can both move on freely and clearly. You don't need the other person in the relationship present, but you could use an energy practitioner or intuitive to help you cut these strong cords or create a ceremony of your own.

Do keep in mind though, that if you continue to have contact with the person (in all forms; texting, speaking, seeing, emailing), the cords redevelop. If possible, no contact for a while is advisable. If that's not possible, in the case of co-parenting for example, you can still do the ceremony to cut the personal relationship cords and then ask the Angels to surround your ex and yourself in your own separate pillars of white light before you know you're going to interact with one another. This is done with the intention to keep your personal feelings Angelically protected and to yourself, so that your interactions are for the highest and best good of the child(ren). And if there's a financial battle in a relationship dissolution, that's its own set of cords. For such a major life change I would suggest a few energetic sessions with a qualified and trusted practitioner to separate the energies and help the parting become more harmonious.

Cleansing an Object

I mentioned earlier that when buying used and new items, you're also taking in the energy of whoever handled it or used it before. So it's a good practice to cleanse all you buy, are gifted, or bring into your home and personal space.

What you'll need:

White sage or Palo Santo or a Cleansing Spray (avoid if working with fabrics)
A lighter, ashtray or fireproof dish

What to do:

Slightly open a window if burning the white sage or palo santo.

Light the sage or palo santo and waft it gently around the object, a few inches away, ensure you have the smoke cover the front, back, sides, above and below the object. If using a spray, spray all around it.

You state your intention by saying these words or use your own
*"I now cleanse this xx (name of object) of all lower energies and
energies not for my highest and greatest good."*

Put out the white sage or palo santo in an ashtray or fireproof dish.

Or, you can call in the Fire Dragons of the Highest Light to cleanse
the object and visualize their fires burning away around the object,
transmuting all lower energies.

Please note: Placing your purse, backpack, or any bag on a public
floor can pick up on lower energies that linger there, which when
you lift your bag up and then hold next to your body, or bring
into your home, transfers on to you and your space. I always try
to place my bag on a chair or keep it on me, and if I have no choice
but to place it on the floor, then I use one of the above methods
to energetically cleanse the bag as soon as I can.

Personal Protection Methods

1. Visualize a White Cocoon of Protection around you. This
   also brings in extra Angels around you.
2. Call upon Archangel Raphael of the Highest Light and ask
   him to place you in a green cocoon of protection around you
   against all germs, bacteria and viruses. I usually do this when
   I'm in large crowds in close proximity.
3. Mirror ball: When you're feeling especially vulnerable, see
   yourself stepping inside a mirrored ball. All negative energy is
   reflected away from the ball.

4. Call upon Archangel Michael of the Highest Light and ask him to place his energetic protection around you. Visualize him placing his blue or purple cocoon of light completely around you and your aura.
5. Ask your personal Dragon to shadow you and use their fire to transmute all negativity headed your way.
6. You can ask the Angels to stand guard in your energetic protection.
   Visualize two Angels standing before you and two behind you as your spiritual bodyguards.
7. Wear a protective crystal on your body. Such as black obsidian, shungite or black tourmaline.
8. If you're in a meeting with someone and you start to feel drained and exhausted, do the following: clasp your hands together by interlacing your fingers and rest them over your solar plexus chakra. Or place a book or your bag over the solar plexus to prevent cords from attaching. You can do this also when on the phone. But still cut the cords after the meeting to be sure.
9. If you walk into a place and realize ugh, this does not feel like a great vibe, and you can't leave, then quickly send a request to Archangel Michael of the Highest Light to place you in an additional shaft of white light. In your minds' eye, see that shaft of white light coming down around you, with you in the middle and connecting into Earth beneath you.

Trust that you are receiving what you asked for.

With all protection, reapply after 4-6 hours depending on where you are. At home, you would not need any or less.

Keep in mind though, that even with protection, we must try to maintain our thoughts, words and actions of a high vibration. If we've asked for protection before leaving the house and then get angry and irritated at the traffic, and start swearing at the other drivers, we attract the same anger and irritation into our energy field. We really need to be quite mindful of how we're feeling and thinking and what we're projecting outwards.

Remember, we are energetic magnets.

Otherwise, we could do and go wherever, with no consequences and just call in our Spiritual team to fix things. But part of our human experience is co-creating our reality and taking responsibility for our actions. We can create positive or negative experiences.

Home Cleansing, Grounding and Protection

Just as you do personally, your home is also a space to be treasured and maintained.

Cleansing

First, physically clean your home, or your own personal space in your home. This means dusting, washing, mopping, vacuuming, etc. and secondly, remove all physical clutter. Dirt and clutter can trap stagnant energy and murky lower energies so this is an essential step.

When cleaning, you can put a sprinkle of sea salt in the mop water which will also clean energetically as you mop. If vacuuming, you can lightly spritz a cleansing spray (recipes to follow) and then vacuum. Or, if the carpet is very delicate and could not withstand liquid at all, sprinkle a tiny bit of sea salt in the four corners of the room and let it sit for 20 minutes and then vacuum it up and empty the vacuum filter and take the garbage out of the house.

To protect yourself from personally absorbing dirty energy in the space, place a smoky quartz crystal in your pocket with the intention it will absorb on your behalf while you clean. Then be sure to cleanse the crystal at the end of the day with the crystal cleansing methods coming up.

Next, use one of the Personal Cleansing and Clearing Methods (page 158-9, numbers 2 or 4 or 5) to clear each room. If using method number 2, be thorough; walking through the home, wafting along each wall, in the corners, behind doors that are normally open, in closets, the ceiling (the smoke will rise naturally) and in doorways. You can just lightly waft, it doesn't need to be a fumigation of smoke.
If using number 4 or 5, visualize the work being done in each room, in every nook and cranny.

Grounding

Altar Space

This is an optional choice, but an Altar is a grounding aspect of a home and it can be as simple or elaborate as you like It's bringing the Divine into your 3D reality. It's not religious but rather an homage to your Soul and its connection to the Universe. You don't need to sit and pray or meditate in front it, although you surely could of course.

It's a personal space that you create wherever you'd like. It's often a shelf at a higher level on the wall, or within a bookcase, or on a corner table, some people might put it in a closet. Somewhere it's not going to be disturbed (the kitchen table or bathroom counter is not ideal) It's a personal choice as to where, although just be mindful that you place it in a safe place if you're going to put a live candle or incense on it. Nothing too close to flammable items! And blow out the candle and incense when you leave the house. Some prefer the battery-operated candles on their altar so it burns always which is also fine.

You can also modify your altar each full moon, or even each week if you prefer. The energy of it does need tending like a garden. Ensure it stays dust free, and clean and cleanse the crystals once a month if you have crystals on it.

Suggested Altar Items (entirely your choice, these are just ideas):

Fabric tablecloth in a colour(s) that resonates with you
White candle (live or battery-operated)
Incense holder for sandalwood, frankincense, myrrh, or oud incense. Whatever scent appeals to you.
Pictures or statues of spiritual Deities/Beings
Pictures of ancestors, or a piece of jewelry owned by an ancestor (to honour your lineage, whatever it may be)
A particular oracle card that resonates with you
Items from nature to represent the elementals and honour Earth (shell, crystal, rock, feather, bowl of water)
Sacred geometric symbols
A written list of things you want to manifest
Crystals that you resonate with

And anything else that has some special meaning to you. There is no right or wrong way, it's your personal Altar!

Protection

1. Ask Archangel Michael of the Highest Light to protect your home each day, asking him to place his Angels at the windows and doors protecting the space and all in it.

   A variation to protect your vehicle each day..as you sit in your car before driving say, *"I ask the Angels and Dragons to protect me and my car and our passengers in a pink bubble of love and light throughout our travels today."*

2. Ask the Dragon Arthur Victorious to place his sentry Dragons to protect your home.

   This can also be done for your vehicle especially if parked in an unsafe area.

3. Another option is to create a Crystal Grid of Protection in the home to energetically protect. Although keep in mind that if you have this grid in place, any Earthbound Spirits who happen to come in with someone's energy will need to be removed up to the light as they won't be able to get out of the grid and leave the space. Homes without a grid, Spirits can come and go.

   Also, if the grid is moved or shaken in any way, then it topples it all so you have to redo it. If you get a lot of traffic through your home and a lot of activity, ensure you strengthen your grid every month or so. I first hired a practitioner to create grids in my home until I learnt how to do it myself. I've explained the steps to create one here.

What you'll need:

6 small crystals (you can choose either black obsidian, tigers' eye, tourmaline, clear quartz, rose quartz)

Blu Tack (also called Sticky Tac, or adhesive putty)
Selenite wand (you can also use your finger)

What to do:

The grid should be placed in a drawer that is never opened, or on a high shelf in a closet, somewhere it's tucked away and unseen and untouched. It only has to take up a small area of space (book or laptop sized), your intention in building it is that it represents and covers the whole home.

Place a bit of the blu tack under each crystal so it sticks to the surface firmly and won't move. Carpet underneath is not ideal as the crystals could slide around.

Place them in the shape of two inverted triangles, a six pointed star, pressing firmly down so the blu tack holds them in place.

With your wand, connect the crystals following the order on the diagram at the end of this book.

Then, once you have connected all six crystals, place your wand at the top again and draw a circle around the whole shape three times.

After three times, lift away your wand and say *"I ask the Angels and Dragons to keep this protective grid in place until I so remove it"*. But as I said, if the crystals move for any reason, the grid needs to be redone.

Practical Energy Tools

In the tools listed below I suggest several items for yourself and the home to help create and maintain a high vibration and clear space.

Candles
A candle is a representation of the Fire Elementals and has a

tremendous energy just within its little flame. Angels love candle flames. Whereas Earthbound Spirits avoid them.

Colours

As mentioned in Chapter 7, each colour has a vibration and will emanate that vibration into a room and on your person. There are also companies who offer coloured non-prescription energy therapy glasses to wear when you want to shift your mood, or enhance a particular one. This is one I know of but I'm sure there are more: www.colourenergy.com

Crystals

Crystals are natural objects coming from the Earth and each type of crystal has its own energetic vibration which can influence a home and person wearing it.

As humans, our vibrations are constantly fluctuating and easily influenced as we're exposed to all the external stimuli around us. Crystals, however, have a very stable energy frequency that doesn't change. More stable energy equals more powerful energy! Powerful energy can influence the energies around it which is how crystals influence our energy and the homes we live in. Each crystal has their own benefits that can help us. There are numerous books and online resources that have information about all the types of crystals and what their benefits are, so I won't list them here, but what I want to focus on is how to care for them once you have them. This includes crystals that are set into jewelry.

As with all things, please be discerning that you are buying them from a reputable place selling the real deal. There are fakes out there.

Cleansing and Preparing Crystals

After receiving the crystal (bought, gifted to you, or found):

1. Clean it physically first. But please check with the store, or a crystal book, on whether the specific crystal likes water. As Selenite for instance, does not do well in water and some fade in prolonged exposure to sunlight. All enjoy a full moon.
The first step is to clean it physically from whoever touched it beforehand. As our fingerprints leave an oily residue. If your crystal is not a water lover, wipe it with a soft clean cloth and place it outside in direct sunlight for ONLY 30 minutes. This is a short enough time for even those that don't prefer sun.
2. Cleanse them energetically. Crystals are live objects and absorb the energy around them. That means energy from everyone who held them before you got them and the space they were in waiting to be selected. Here you have several options;
"I ask this sacred smoke to energetically cleanse this crystal." Burn white sage or palo santo around each individual crystal.
"I ask the great central sun to energetically cleanse this crystal." Place in direct sunlight.
"I ask Mother Earth and the Earth Elementals to please energetically cleanse this crystal." Place them on earth/dirt in the garden/ sand at the beach/on the grass for at least 4 hours.

Once you bring the cleansed crystal back indoors, set the intention you'd like it to help you with. An intention is like anchoring your desired goals to the crystal's stable power.
For example, for a rose quartz pendant, hold it in your dominant hand and you could say *"bring more self-love into my life."*
For an amethyst that you have on a table at home, *"help me connect to the Spiritual realm during my meditation or contemplation."*

This is why it's good to know the specific properties of each crystal you have. And if you don't have a specific request you can always say, holding it, *"I ask this crystal to help align me with my greatest and highest good."*

Please note that **monthly maintenance** to cleanse all your crystals is very important. Your crystals will absorb your energy, the energy of your home and whoever's in it. So for them to generate their power optimally, place them outside in the full moon overnight each month. If it's freezing cold temperatures or you find some sneaky nocturnal animals are running off with some of the crystals (it's happened!), you can place them in the window sill the night of a full moon. Set the intention *"I ask the power and light of the full moon to cleanse all of these crystals and recharge their power."*

Energy Sprays
Also called Aura Sprays. Used to cleanse the energy in a space or around a person. Or to bring in a desired beneficial energy. Most holistic stores and Etsy have a variety to choose from, and you can also make your own. I've included a few recipes here but you can also research the benefits of oils you like and create your own.

Energy Spray Recipes

Clearing spray
For home and personal use

6-8 drops Sage essential oil (can also use camphor, eucalyptus, rosemary. Choose one, do not blend)
Distilled water
Witch Hazel or any type of clear alcohol (this is to preserve the spray over time)

A dash of sea salt

120 ml/4 oz glass or plastic bottle (I prefer glass but it's not as easy to find so you can use plastic too)

First fill the bottle 90% full of distilled water. Then drop the sage essential oil in. The more drops, the stronger the smell, not necessarily a stronger spray. Sprinkle in the sea salt. Fill the remaining 10% of your preservative choice (witch hazel, rubbing alcohol, clear flavourless vodka). Place the nozzle on the bottle and give it a shake.

Set the intention:

In front of a candle, holding the bottle in both hands, state, *"I decree that this energy spray will clear all negative and lower energies under Grace in a perfect way wherever I spray it."*

Added bonus:

Place the bottle outside overnight during a full moon to charge it. If it's winter with freezing temperatures, place it on a windowsill and state, *"I ask the energy and power of the full moon tonight to charge this energy spray with the highest cleansing energies and capacity to clear."*

Confidence builder spray

For personal use

6-8 drops Valor™ Young Living essential oil blend (or Doterra Balance™ blend)

OR you can blend your own variety of oils from some or all of the below:

Frankincense essential oil

Geranium essential oil

Sandalwood essential oil

Cedarwood essential oil
Lavender essential oil

Distilled water
Witch Hazel or any type of clear alcohol
120ml/4 oz glass or plastic bottle
Optional: Tiny crystal chips/pieces of Tigers Eye crystal, or one small piece of Tigers Eye that fits into the bottle neck. Tigers Eye provides confidence and courage and will infuse the spray with its own properties, making it a more powerful spray.

First fill the bottle 90% full of distilled water. Then drop the essential oils in. Insert the crystals if you have them. Fill the remaining 10% of your preservative choice. Place the nozzle on the bottle and give it a shake.

Set the intention:
In front of a candle, holding the bottle in both hands, state *"I decree that this energy spray will bring in more confidence and courage under Grace in a perfect way on whoever uses it."*

Added bonus:
Place the bottle outside overnight during a full moon to charge it. *"I ask the energy and power of the full moon tonight to charge this energy spray with the highest energy of confidence and courage."*

Abundance spray
For home and personal use

Abundance™ Young Living essential oil blend
OR you can blend your own variety of oils from some or all of the below:

Frankincense
Myrrh
Orange
Lemon

Distilled water
Witch Hazel or any type of clear alcohol
120 ml/4 oz glass or plastic bottle
Optional: Tiny crystal chips/pieces of Citrine crystal, or one small piece of Citrine that fits into the bottle neck. Citrine is an abundance attractor and will infuse the spray with its own properties, making it a more powerful spray.

First fill the bottle 90% full of distilled water. Then drop the essential oils in. Insert the crystals if you have them. Fill the remaining 10% of your preservative choice. Place the nozzle on the bottle and give it a shake.

Set the intention:
In front of a candle, and holding the bottle in both hands, state *"I decree that this energy spray will bring in more financial abundance under Grace in a perfect way on whoever uses it."*

Added bonus:
Place the bottle outside overnight during a full moon to charge it. *"I ask the energy and power of the full moon tonight to charge this energy spray with the highest energy of financial and wealth abundance."*

Please note: Young Living and Doterra are oils that I've used but you can use any other quality essential oil in your sprays.

Essential Oil Diffusers

These are machines used to disperse the aroma of an essential oil into a room. A practice of Aromatherapy, diffusers can use heat, water, or an atomizer to spread the scent into the room. Not as an air freshener, but for actually changing the vibration of the room by infusing it with the qualities of the essential oils. A calmer atmosphere, use lavender. Studying or using mental faculties, use peppermint. Essential oils are not good for most pets so I don't advise using them if you have them in the house.

Incense

This aromatic essence comes in a variety of forms, either as long sticks (most common), cones, coils, wood pieces (oud for instance). They either burn themselves once lit, or can be placed on hot coals and smolder from that heat source. All release an aromatic smoke into the air. The incense itself are originally made with plant-based ingredients and can include a variety of resins, barks, seeds, roots, flowers and sometimes added essential oils. However today many are made with synthetic materials that are cheaper to produce.

It's been used traditionally for centuries in offerings, prayers, honouring the spiritual world, warding off negative entities, and combating medieval odours. Today, you'll see it in yoga studios, shops, offices, homes. There is no real rule of where you can and can't burn incense. Choose a scent you like and use it as a home air cleanser, on your altar to honour the Air Elementals, during a ceremony, or whenever the mood takes you. Just be sure to use a holder to catch all the ash that comes off as it burns, as it can burn the surface it sits on.

White Sage

This is an herb that is dried and tied up into a bundle, for burning to clear a space, object or person of negative energies. There are many different varieties of Sage and the one used for Smudging (clearing a space of negative energies) is called White Sage. A little different to the one you cook with and buy at the grocery store. However, I have lived in places where it was hard to buy white sage and I used the cooking variety as a substitute that also worked.

Please note: Some say Smudging will remove Earthbound Spirits and it may repel them for a while, but once the smoke clears, they could come back. Sage is best used for dissipating negative energies.

How to use it:

Optional: Call in Archangel Michael of the Highest Light and his clearing Angels to help you clear with this sage.

With a lighter, light up one end of a bundle. (Sage is normally sold in bundles). You may want to hold a little smudge bowl or an ashtray underneath to catch the burning embers which fall off. With one hand holding the bowl/ashtray, and the other holding the lit sage bundle...

To cleanse a home - Open a window, walk around the perimeter of each room in a house wafting the sage along the walls, floors, corners, behind doors, in closets.

To cleanse an object - Open a window, waft the sage around all sides, top and bottom of the object, allowing the smoke to clear the energy.

To cleanse a vehicle - Doors open, waft the sage through all parts of the interior, trunk, outside body.

To cleanse a person or yourself - Open a window, waft the sage around your body, all sides, behind you, in front of you, above your head, beneath your feet, under your armpits, between your legs.

Remember to watch out for burning embers that may fall off and burn the floor/surroundings if you don't have the dish underneath.

Once completed, let it burn out in the dish, or stamp it lightly out in the dish, or place it under running water to put it out.

Palo Santo

Another aromatic essence used for cleansing. Palo Santo comes from a sacred tree indigenous to Central and South America and is used much like white sage as a cleanser of negative energies. It comes as little sticks and you hold one lit end while wafting it around what you're cleansing. Both produce the same effect so it's your preference on what to use.

You can follow the same directions from White Sage on how to use Palo Santo.

You may not need a dish underneath but an ash will form so you may need to tap it off every so often. You also may need to lightly blow on the Palo Santo stick to keep the embers burning.

Once completed, let it burn out in the dish or place it under running water to put it out.

Please note: Because Palo Santo has become so popular worldwide, I suggest researching who and where you buy from to ensure its ethically sourced and also the real thing, and not just pieces of wood with synthetic scent added to it. The spiritual essence of Palo Santo (which means holy wood in Spanish) comes from the Bursera graveolens tree branches that have naturally broken off, or a tree that has naturally fallen or died before the Palo Santo can be harvested from it. Because otherwise, we're using an item to cleanse for higher vibrations from a tree that we are taking its wood, its essence, without permission.

Here is one company that ethically sources, and there are others as well: https://animamundiherbals.com/collections/all/products/palo-santo-sacred-wood-incense

All herbs (including White Sage) we use should really be harvested in a respectful way, asking permission of the plant to cut and remove. But unless you do it yourself, this is difficult to be aware of.

Sea Salt

Sea salt has very powerful purification and protection qualities. This is salt produced by evaporation of ocean water or water from salt-water lakes. It's less processed than iodized table salt. For spiritual uses, use only sea salt or Himalayan pink salt. The purest forms of salt. Salt is a crystal so it absorbs energy. Some cultures place salt at the entrance to homes aand around beds as protection, and here are a few other suggestions on how to use it...

1. In an energy spray to cleanse
2. In the water when cleaning the floor
3. If you're a practitioner working with other's energies, place a bowl of salt water near you during the sessions (tap water and a few tablespoons of salt). Ask the salt and Water Elementals to absorb all negative energies in your area. When you finish

working, thank the Elementals and flush the salt water down the toilet.

4. In a sea salt bath. 2 cups in your bathtub and soak for minimum 20 minutes.

Himalayan Salt Lamps

This is based on Halotherapy and range from small to larger chunks of pink/orange salt with a hole in the middle and a corded small wattage lightbulb in the centre. They're mined from Pakistan's northern Punjab region at the Khewra Salt Mine. This salt can also come as a food seasoning, as candle holders, bricks, and more. Placing one or more of these lamps in your home can provide the following benefits:

- Neutralizes EMF radiation (from phones, Wi-Fi, Bluetooth, TV's, computers, etc.)
- Purifies, refreshes and enhances air quality
- Improves breathing
- Has a relaxing effect

They're meant to always be turned on with a low wattage (4 or 7w bulb). If they're not on and you live in a humid environment, the salt lamp can 'leak' and you'll find crusty salt water deposits below. I personally have one in each room of my house.

Halotherapy (Salt Therapy)

Since the 19th century, salt treatment caves have been used in therapeutic settings to help those with respiratory problems. In the 1980's, a Halotherapy device called the Halogenerator which grinds pure salt particles and releases it into the room, was invented for those who didn't have access to a salt cave. Nowadays, this treatment has spread across the world with the creation of Salt Caves built within a storefront, for people to visit, sit, and enjoy the benefits of Himalayan Salt. Usually the room is built from large salt bricks, surrounding you in thousands of pounds of Himalayan salt with the Halogenerator grinding the salt particles and releasing them into the cave. A place to heal, revive, relax, meditate and breathe.

Protection against EMF Radiation (Electromagnetic Field)

As we've discussed earlier, most natural environments outside have a balanced harmonious energy with cleaner air and positive energy flowing. But in more densely populated areas that are full of cell phone towers, microwaves, radio waves, Wi-Fi, Bluetooth, and so on, these all emit EMF radiation and can affect living beings in a negative way. Everyone may have different ranges of sensitivity to it, but these EMF waves in the air can create stressful energy. Which in turn can lead to our own energy being imbalanced, our animals being affected, even the plants in our home. The following items are a few things you can use in your home to negate the effects of EMF. You can even go a step further and purchase an EMF Meter to really check what areas of your home are bombarding you and your family, and therefore, where to place these items.

Orgonite

These are often created in the shape of pyramids, but can also be any other shape and even made into pendants. It's a manmade item that consists of resin, metals, and a crystal that when combined, balance the energy around it. Some also add sacred geometric symbols to increase the healing frequencies. The Orgonite absorbs the unbalanced energy by the metal-resin mix and is brought back to a healthier positive state by the crystal.

Place the Orgonite wherever you have the most EMF radiation in your home, or with a plant, or outside with your garden (ensure it's made for outdoor use in that case).

Copper
Copper is one of the most effective metals to block and shield EMF radiation because of its ability to reduce the force of magnetic and electrical waves.

Aluminum Foil is also a good method to block EMF radiation, remember the tin foil hats the conspiracy theorists are accused of wearing? Not so fantastical. While it's not that aesthetically pleasing to line your home with aluminum foil, there are companies who offer copper products to place in your home, on yourself (as a pendant), and your cell phone (as a disc) to shield from harmful effects of EMF.

Place the copper directly in between you and the source of EMF radiation (for example, the Wi-Fi modem in your home).

Crystals
From experience, I found placing a very large grounding crystal near a Wi-Fi modem can help lessen the effects too.
I used to get such an anxious feeling while watching TV and I couldn't figure out why. It wasn't the content, light hearted comedies usually. (My Wi-Fi modem happens to sit beside the TV.) When I placed a large chunk of black obsidian (it's about 7" in height and 4" in depth) crystal on a shelf beneath the modem, it helped enormously. No more anxiety if I was near the modem. That little box emits some strong signals. I don't have an EMF meter but I had ear buds in while listening to my phone and when I was by the modem, the sound got all crackly and broken up and improved when I moved away from it.

In general, it's best to keep your bed away from as many electronics as you can so you can get a restful night's sleep. If you must have your phone beside you as a clock or alarm, turn it to airplane mode while you sleep.

Wind Chimes

These are a type of percussion instrument often made of metal or wood suspended from the ceiling with tubes, rods, bells or other objects. When the natural movement of air goes through the objects, it creates its own tinkling sound, depending on what it's made of. The ancient reason for using them was to attract good spirits.

When the wind moves the metal, wood, or whatever your chimes are made of, it disperses stagnant energy thereby purifying and enhancing energy within a certain area. It's not something you'd remove and walk around with, it's a stationary piece within your home, usually in the garden/patio/balcony.

Evil Eye Protection

This symbol is often worn as an amulet or pendant hanging in a home or on your person. You may even see it painted on an airplane today for protection. This symbol is very ancient, dating as far back as 5000BC in Mesopotamia (modern day Iraq, Kuwait, Turkey and Syria). It was used to ward of curses or malicious intent. The symbol wards off the negativity from *the* evil eye, which was a curse transmitted through a malicious glare, usually inspired by envy.

Sometimes you see it within a 'Hamsa' which is a symbol of an open palm (the Hand of God) with the evil eye nesting within, offering dual protection, blessing, and good fortune.

More commonly, the eye design is portrayed as a single eye in blue, black and white hues. Sometimes as a full eye, sometimes stylized as a single dot on a background to represent the pupil and the iris. And almost always against a blue background, a protective colour. It can be worn as jewelry for personal protection, or hung opposite a door at the entrance of a home.

Plants, Fresh Flowers

These items in a home always freshen up the air and energy of the space. They're living organisms which emanate their own aura and energy. Peaceful and calm from healthy plants. Flowers and plants can help improve the flow of positive energy in a home, purify the air and increase a sense of well-being. You can also invite and thank the Earth Elementals into your home through your live plants, as well as ask them for help in maintaining healthy growth.

Vision Boards

These are visual representations of your hopes, dreams, desires and goals. The point is to create them with pictures, words, colours, and symbols, in whatever way resonates with you, so that when your gaze lands on it on a daily basis, you feel excitement, hope, expectation of the realization of these goals. It's not a shopping list to the Universe or so simple that if you put a picture of a Ferrari on it you'll magically get one. It's more that the image of the Ferrari may represent abundance, freedom, Italy, sleekness, design, craftsmanship, beauty. Viewing that car on your board produces *the emotions* within you.

You could also personalize the pictures, for instance, when I wanted to move to a different province, I found a picture of what their drivers license looked like and glued a picture of my face on the driving license and placed that on my vision board. Representing that I wanted to move to that province, be a resident and have a vehicle and I got excited whenever I glanced at it. I also had a picture of a car with my photo in the drivers seat. I still had to do the work and take steps to move, but I was letting the universe know my intention as well. Just glancing at my board would prompt me to daydream and imagine living there. Emanating the energy of what I wanted to manifest.

Think of this as a creative way to set goals.

You can find a great deal of information online about vision boards but it's really something you create that makes you smile, opens your heart, and prompts a positive emotional reaction within you.

How to make a Vision Board

What you'll need:

A poster board or large sheet of paper. It can be as large and as thick as you want it, I like to use the poster boards from the $1 store.
Images and/or phrases cut out from magazines, photos, postcards or printed from the internet
Glue or clear tape
A candle
A permanent marker
Any other crafts you want to add (it could be glitter, stickers, dried flowers - this is YOUR creation and can look however you want).

How to make it:

Light your candle and state out loud or in your head what your intention is in creating this vision board. (To manifest, to create a vibe, an energy of how you'd like your reality to be, etc.)

At the top of your board write in the centre with the marker, "All this or something even better"

And then...use your own intuition and creativity to cut out the images and/or words or phrases you want on your board. You can lay it out first and then glue or tape these to your board in whatever way speaks to you. You could add glitter or stickers or decorative items in the corners and in between, or just leave it as images. You are the artist with this canvas.

Once you're finished, place both hands over the board blessing it with love and excitement that this is on its way to you.

Blow out the candle.

Place your board in a place that you'll see it every day, the idea is when your eyes land on it, it will fill you with the warm and fuzzies, giving you a ping of excitement that those visions are coming to life. If you share your home with others and prefer to keep your board private, hang it on the inside of a closet or wardrobe door so only you see it every morning when you get your clothes for the day.

There are also apps that allow you to create a digital vision board, and some people prefer to cut and paste images digitally onto their board. That's fine too, but ensure you print it out large so you can see it often. No point to create it for it to stay buried on your phone or computer. Unless you actively open the app and look at it each day.

Journaling
This is writing down your thoughts and feelings to release them or understand them more clearly. Writing freely, only for yourself,

without judgement by anyone ever reading it. There are no specific tips or guidelines, it's simply writing what you're feeling and thinking so you don't bottle anything negative down internally. Which eventually bubbles to the surface and explodes, maybe not right away, could be years and years from now, or you may even carry it into the next lifetime as lessons to overcome.

You can choose any notebook if you prefer to write by hand, or a journaling app, or a text document on your computer or phone. Write with abandon, don't worry about spelling or punctuation. You can always re-read it later but that's not necessary. The practice is more about getting it all out to release it.

Writing Letters

A faction of journaling is writing letters to individuals at the end of relationships, people who've hurt you, anyone who you feel anger, resentment or unforgiveness towards. You do this to help yourself move on and let go. You may have to write more than one letter, and you never send it. Your burn it, or rip it up and throw it away to symbolically release the emotions. Try to balance the letter with all the things you never said and what you're angry about, but also put a little positivity in it, like "Thank you for teaching me that I need to set my boundaries stronger" or, "thanks for the good times, the fun". By ending the letter this way, perhaps a little sliver of forgiveness can come into your heart. If you still feel immense hatred or anger after writing it, keep doing it until those feelings lessen. It may take more than one. And it may take weeks, months or even years before you really feel a shift. But with your intention and action, and asking your Spiritual team to help you release, a shift will indeed come.

Manifesting

Manifesting is about taking control of your thoughts, words and actions and putting steps into place that will help you reach your goal. It's calling in the energy and being a vibrational match to it. However, we cannot forget that our Soul has it's own individual agreements and contracts that it agreed to before reincarnation that cannot be avoided. It's not everyone's path to be billionaires, otherwise we'd all be one! Our manifesting can bring us what we need and what is for our highest and best purpose.

Creating vision boards, writing life scripts, making lists, visualizations, mantras, affirmations, guided meditations, are all various methods that can help and there are many resources with further information on manifestation techniques. Use whatever resonates with you and then LET IT GO. You don't need to share your intended manifestations with anyone else either, instead, nurture it like a tiny seedling that you plant. Unless someone has a direct involvement with your actions to manifest, then there's no need to announce it to other people. You're shielding and protecting it from energies that may be full of disbelief and opinions that are from others projections and belief systems and nothing to do with your capabilities and skills.

Once you let it go, you can continue to do the energy work to heal and release past issues and wounds so that you become clearer mentally and emotionally with more capacity to enjoy all these wonderful things that are about to come into your life!

Oracle Cards
We discussed these in Chapter 6, so I'll be brief here and just point out that these are nice little tools to connect with the Spiritual realm every day. With a deck of your choice, shuffle while asking the question *"what's the guidance for me today"* or *"what do I need to be aware of today"*. And then when it feels right, pull one card for

your answer.

You can also use this tool to ask more specific questions regarding what's going on in your life at the moment.

Please note, when you purchase an Oracle card deck, they should be energetically cleared. Then you should sit with them, holding them, going through each card, touching them with your hands, charging it with your energy. When not in use, keep them in a safe place. If someone else handles your cards, you'll want to do the cleansing and charging process again to get it in tune with your energy once more.

Prayer

Prayer can be a lot of different things to different people and done in a myriad of ways. If it resonates with you, prayer is a nice way to connect and speak with the Divine and ask for what you need. You could use established traditional words or your own words, imagine it's like picking up the phone and connecting to God and the telephone line is then buzzing with the energy between you two. You could also pray for the well-being of others and places; your words and intentions do have an effect on the collective consciousness.

Why do we need to know all this?

As you've learned, humans are complex, multi-sensory beings with a constant inner connection to the Spiritual realm. Everything we think, feel, say or do has an effect on our lives. What we read, watch, listen to, and talk about has an effect on our lives. Who we spend the majority of our time with influences our lives. And how we take care of our physical, emotional, mental and spiritual selves can transform our lives for the positive, or the negative. We have so much responsibility for our well-being, and we rarely feel or realize the magnitude of our own personal power.

Because that's what this is. The information in this book is to help you realize your personal power to create a life you want. Sure, there may be Soul challenges to overcome that you can't change, but by facing them, defeating them, and then healing and letting go, you can stop those karmic cycles to fix the same problem lifetime after lifetime. And to help you in this quagmire, are a whole team of Spiritual Beings just waiting for you to ask them for help. It's never too late to shift things, to reclaim your true self. Shed all the old belief systems, the traumas, the cords, the energetic imprints that are just dragging you down or keeping you stagnant. It's time to move forward with Light, Love, Confidence, Hope and Faith.

Faith in yourself first and foremost.

The Next Steps in your Magical Journey

You're ready! You can incorporate all the tools, or one, or none. Perhaps the knowledge you've gained is enough to shift your mindset and energy. You are all beautiful, unique individuals on your own path and you must do what's right for you.

Here are a few highlights to remember during daily life...

- Stay mindful of your thoughts, feelings, words and actions. They hold tremendous power.
- Connect daily. To your Higher Self, and/or your Spiritual team.
- Meditate daily or set aside time for stillness and silence.
- Physically ensure you are always grounded, nourishing your body with high quality food & drink, and moving your body in some way regularly.

- Get outside as often as you can.
- Cleanse your energy daily using whatever method you prefer.
- Protect your energy daily using whatever method you prefer.
- In relationships (whether family, friends, colleagues, clients), remember you can't change anyone, you can only change your reaction. Don't take anything personally.
- It's okay to set loving boundaries. Your self-care first.
- Anything you bring into your home is bringing its past energy and the energy of whoever handled it. Clear the objects using whatever method you prefer.
- Same as with your vehicle. Particularly if other people are driving it, or servicing it.

It's never too late to remedy your course and improve, adjust, and bring balance to your life once again. Everything can be fixed and healed. You just need to dedicate the time and self-care to yourself and ask for the help you need.

The 21 Day Program

Helping You on Your Journey

This is not a diet or exercise program but focuses more on your Spiritual Self to help you get into a practice of mindfulness, self-awareness, connection, inner balance and healing.

The best way to take mastery of your energy and space is to implement a daily practice. Like showering or brushing your teeth, this can be as little or as long a process as you like. It may seem daunting at first but after some time, it'll feel so natural and if you miss a day, you'll feel like something is missing. By doing this, you're keeping yourself and your surroundings' vibration high, for your own well-being and also for your Spiritual team to connect easier.

This program is gentle, with mainly a time commitment from your side. You don't have to immediately go buy oracle cards, statues or anything like that. Right now, the intent is for you to connect to yourself first and then you can use tools that resonate with you later on.

These 21 days are suggestions for those who like to follow a guideline with specific steps. You can also create your own 21 day program, the key is consistence EACH DAY and for the full 21 days. You're creating new habits, new energies and releasing the old. So, it's important to keep up the momentum with discipline.

All meditations in the Program can be found for free on my YouTube channel.

Preparation for the Program

Finish reading this book so everything you're doing makes more sense.

Buy a journal, or download a journal app. Day One is an app that I use, but there are many more to choose from.

Buy some White Sage, or Palo Santo or an energy spray (or make your own).

WEEK 1: CLEAR

This week we're starting the process to clear and shift your own energies and the energy in your immediate surroundings.

Day 1: AM:
1. While you're still in bed, using your journal, make a note of the mood you woke up in, or the thought that first came into your head. Without judgement, just as a recording of it. It doesn't have to be long, it could be a sentence or even just a word.
2. Throughout the day, pay attention to what you're reading, watching and listening to. And who you're interacting with. Make a note of it in your journal. How do you feel afterwards?

PM: Listen to the Archangel Michael Clearing Meditation (7 minutes) before sleep.

Day 2: AM:
1. While you're still in bed, make a note of your mood/thought first thing.
2. Listen to the Morning Meditation - Centering yourself (7 minutes).
3. Throughout the day, pay attention to what you're reading, watching and listening to. And who you're interacting with. Make a note of it in your journal. How do you feel afterwards?
Did the morning meditation make a difference in your day?
PM: Listen to the Archangel Michael Clearing Meditation (7 minutes) before sleep.

Day 3: AM:
1. While you're still in bed, make a note of your mood/thought first thing.
2. Listen to the Morning Meditation - Infusing your day with Joy (8 minutes).
3. Throughout the day, pay attention to what you're reading, watching and listening to. And who you're interacting with. Make a note of it in your journal. How do you feel afterwards?
Did the morning meditation make a difference in your day?
PM: Listen to the Archangel Michael Clearing Meditation (7 minutes) before sleep.

Day 4: AM:
1. While you're still in bed, make a note of your mood/thought first thing.
2. Listen to the Boost your Confidence Meditation (16 minutes).
3. Throughout the day, pay attention to what you're reading,

watching and listening to. And who you're interacting with. Make a note of it in your journal. How do you feel afterwards?

Did the morning meditation make a difference in your day?

PM: Listen to Raising your Vibration Meditation (36 minutes) before sleep (it's okay if you fall asleep while listening).

Day 5: AM:

1. While you're still in bed, make a note of your mood/thought first thing.

2. Throughout the day, pay attention to what you're reading, watching and listening to. And who you're interacting with. Make a note of it in your journal. How do you feel afterwards?

PM:

1. Take a Sea Salt bath, or use sea salt as a scrub in the shower.

2. Listen to Raising your Vibration Meditation (36 minutes) before sleep.

Day 6: AM: This day is best done whenever you have a free day with more time.

1. While you're still in bed, make a note of your mood/thought first thing.

2. Listen to the Alignment Meditation (16 minutes).

3. Physically clean and remove/reduce clutter of your home/space/vehicle.

4. Use your choice of the White Sage/Palo Santo/Energy Spray to cleanse your home/room,   vehicle and self.

5. Choose a protection method from Chapter 8 for yourself and your home/room/vehicle.

PM: Listen to Raising your Vibration Meditation (36 minutes) before sleep.

Day 7: AM:

1. While you're still in bed, make a note of your mood/thought first thing.

2. Review the past seven days of your recorded moods and thoughts. Are they the same?

Were there any shifts either positive or negative?

How would you like to change them?

Start a fresh page in your journal titled 'My Intention for the upcoming week' and list how you'd like to improve upon your waking thoughts and mood. It can be bullet points, a few words, or pages long, up to you. Just set that intention for the coming week.

If you always woke up feeling great and positive, well done you! If that's the case, please still set an intention in the coming week of how you can spread Angelic healing to the world. Each morning, simply ask out loud, or in your mind, *"I send Angels of the Highest Light to surround xx (state the person, country, industry or group (school board, political group, corporation, etc.) today with the highest Divine light of love, healing, wisdom and compassion".*

3. Review from your journal how you felt during the week from what was surrounding you, be it people, places, entertainment, or the news.

If there was a predominance of negative, beneath the 'intentions for the upcoming week' write 'intentions of what I can do to lessen those negative impacts'. Is it less news, more mellow music, more light hearted programs, more time for self-care, less time with certain people? Remember your boundaries!

But go easy on yourself, I'm not asking you to change completely overnight, a little step here and there will still facilitate improvements over time. We are human, and sometimes we go forward, then step back, then go forward. We do the best we can.

4. Sometime during the day, go outside and spend some time in nature. Walking, or any physical activity, or simply sitting outside in silence.

PM: Listen to Raising your Vibration Meditation (36 minutes) before sleep.

Optional:
Book a session this week for an energy clearing and balancing. Distance sessions work just as effectively as in person. You can book one with me, or someone else you resonate with. It's important for you to feel comfortable with whomever you choose. The purpose of this session is to clear and balance a deeper level of your energies and bodies. So that you can operate with more discernment of being your true self without being influenced by other energies or imprints you're carrying.

WEEK 2: CONNECT

This week you're going to start becoming more aware of who and what Beings, guidance, and assistance are around you.

Day 1: AM:
1. As soon as you wake up, start a gratitude practice. These are sample words but you can use your own instead. Always follow your own heart.

"God, (or you can say Universe if you prefer), thank you for this day, thank you for this life, thank you for everything I have and everything I am"

2. Throughout the day continue to be mindful of who you spend

time with, what you listen to, read or watch. And observe how it affects your energy, record any notable moments in your journal. Did you experience a trigger? Did you experience a strong almost overwhelming feeling of anger or sadness to someone? Record it in your journal, and remember to cut the cords at the end of the day.

PM: Go for a walk outside (just 15 minutes if it's cold out! Bundle up and dress warm). Or sit in your backyard/balcony if you have one. Be silent, without music, or anyone else speaking to you, and in your mind, send your greetings to the nature Beings, something like, (or use your own words) *"Hello Mother Nature, the Sun, the Moon, the Earth, Air, Fire and Water Elementals. Thank you for the bounty you give us"*. If you're an early bird, you can also start the day with the walk outside.

These Beings are just doing their thing, minding their own business, but when they hear you speaking to them, acknowledging and thanking them, their little ears prick up and they start to pay attention, like "hmmm..this human knows about us, let's see where this relationship can go".

PM: Listen to Meet your Guardian Angel Meditation (24 minutes) before sleep. Please stay awake for this. Make a note of what information you received during this meditation in your journal.

Day 2: AM:

1. As soon as you wake up, do your gratitude practice.

2. Say hello or good morning, some greeting to your Guardian Angel. As if they're sitting on the end of your bed, or behind it, or sitting on a chair near it. Visualize them near you.

3. Throughout the day continue to be mindful of who you spend time with, what you listen, read or watch. And observe how it affects your energy, record any notable moments in your journal.

PM: Write in your journal to your Guardian Angel, expressing what you'd like to manifest in your life. At the end of the list or script write, *"All this or something even better"*.

Optional: Listen to Bring in the Christ Consciousness Energy meditation (15 minutes), its okay if you fall asleep.

Day 3: AM:
1. As soon as you wake up, do your gratitude practice.
2. Greet your Guardian Angel.
3. Throughout the day continue to be mindful of who you spend time with, what you listen, read or watch. And observe how it affects your energy, record any notable moments in your journal.
The purpose of this repeated mindfulness is to identify, and then eliminate or reduce the factors in your life that contribute to a negative or bleak outlook and energy.
PM: Address your Ancestors tonight. Even if you have no idea who they might be, this process honours them automatically. They will feel it.

In an area where you can be undisturbed, light a candle.
If you have family photos, you can place them beside the candle, or use another object to represent your lineage. It could be a crystal, a flower, a feather, a piece of jewelry owned by one of them, use whatever represents them to you.
Sit in front of these items, close your eyes and either out loud or in your mind, acknowledge your ancestors, saying these words (or use your own, remember it's the intention behind it)
"I honour and acknowledge my ancestors through my paternal and maternal lines, in all dimensions and directions of time. I thank them for the strengths and blessings they've bestowed upon me, and I forgive them for any unresolved karma and patterns. I ask for their help now in this lifetime of mine, to help me release and end all unresolved

karma and burdens so that we are all released from these ties that bind. And so it is. Thank you."

You can visualize energy going back to them, or perhaps you'll sense them near you. Whatever you experience, trust they received and felt this message and intention.

Optional: Listen to Bring in the Christ Consciousness Energy meditation (15 minutes).

Day 4: AM:

1. As soon as you wake up, do your gratitude practice.

2. Greet your Guardian Angel and your Ancestors.

3. Throughout the day continue to be mindful of who you spend time with, what you listen, read or watch. And observe how it affects your energy, record any notable moments in your journal.

PM:

1. Go outside for 15 minute (longer if you're able to), walking in silence, or sitting in silence within nature, greeting the Elementals, Dragon Elementals and Mother Nature as you do so.

2. Listen to Meet your Personal Dragon Meditation (13 minutes), please stay awake for this. Make a note of what information you received during this meditation in your journal.

Day 5: AM:

1. As soon as you wake up, do your gratitude practice.

2. Greet your Guardian Angel, your Ancestors, your Personal Dragon.

3. Throughout the day continue to be mindful of who you spend time with, what you listen, read or watch. And observe how it affects your energy, record any notable moments in your journal.

PM:

1. In your journal, make a list of 3 things you'd like to manifest and

create in your life. Not so much as material goods but more along the lines of personal development. For example;
- release all the emotional burdens I carry from the past which only weigh me down
- receive guidance on the best health choices I can make for myself
- discover my passion as it applies to my life purpose

After you have your list, light a candle, and say
"I call in all of my highest Spiritual guidance and assistance available to me now to help me achieve these intentions. I am now willing and ready to receive and understand your guidance and help. Thank you."
You may close your eyes to feel, sense what comes in, or just start writing ideas, words, anything that pops into your mind. If nothing comes in, not to worry, it'll come in the next hours or days in various ways. Through words you hear, emails out of the blue, a visual, a song, a dream, an animal. There is no limit to how the Spirit world communicates with us. Just stay alert to what surrounds you in the coming days.
2. Listen to Meet your Spiritual Team Meditation, please stay awake. Journal any impressions, messages, names, descriptions of beings, that came through.

Day 6: AM:
1. As soon as you wake up, do your gratitude practice.
2. Greet your Guardian Angel, your Ancestors, your Personal Dragon and your Spirit Guides.
3. Go outside, for a longer time period, an hour if you can. For a walk, or sitting, or any activity. Greet and thank Mother Earth and all the Elementals. You may want to bring your journal along and just fill it with whatever fills you today. It could be more gratitude, complaints, worries, hope, just let it flow out of you, get it all off

your chest and mind. Notice any animals that unusually cross your path. For instance, a squirrel might be common to see, but if you unusually see a bald eagle, flying or sitting, take notice and look up the meaning afterwards.

PM: Listen to Bringing Light into your DNA and Earth mediation (18 minutes) before sleep.

Day 7: AM:

1. As soon as you wake up, do your gratitude practice.

2. Greet your Guardian Angel, your Ancestors, your Personal Dragon and your Spirit Guides.

3. Today, review your journal entries of the past week and observe how you felt, what came through, how did you do with your stated intentions from the beginning of the week?

Would you like to shift your intentions of the coming week ahead? Perhaps one intention could be to shift your reaction to a co-worker, or a family member. And that could be by having a non-reaction instead. So that you remain in peace and not be drawn into drama or an altercation.

Was something distracting you from TV or online? Perhaps you could make an intention to spend less time watching and surfing and go outside more.

Of course, have fun and enjoy life, just try to always have a balance within you - mental, emotional, physical and spiritual.

PM: You have a Spiritual team always communicating with you, and you also have your Higher Self communicating with you.

Practice the Visualization to bring in your Higher Self from Chapter 1.

Do you notice a difference in feeling and energy from your other Spiritual team?

Ask your Higher Self a question about your life. See what image, word, feeling, or knowing comes in gently after you ask. If you don't sense anything, ask your Higher Self to give you a stronger answer later or while you sleep.

You can keep practicing this visualization every day until you start to recognize your Higher Self's 'voice' which is usually very similar to your own thoughts. But I can't say that's the norm because everyone perceives differently.

Optional:

Create your personal Altar.

WEEK 3: BRINGING IT ALL TOGETHER

This week you're going to implement a little daily routine to bring it all together. You can of course amend the routine afterwards, according to what resonates with you, but I just ask for seven days, do the below and then continue on with a daily routine, the same, or adjusted for your preferences.

Day 1 through 7: AM:
Morning routine:
(which can be done lying in bed or with a cup of your morning beverage sitting somewhere you'll be undisturbed. It doesn't take more than 5 minutes, but you can extend it for longer meditation, prayer, specific requests)

1. Connect with your body, ground into Mother Earth. See Chapter 8 for details.
2. Bring in and connect with your Higher Self. Breathe here for a few minutes.

3. Express your gratitude. And, if it resonates, you can say a prayer such as:

"Dear God, I give this day to you. May my mind stay centered on the things of Spirit. May I not be tempted to stray from love. As I begin this day, I open to receive You. Please enter where You already abide. May my mind and heart be pure and true, and may I not deviate from the things of goodness. Amen. (1)"
OR
"Dear God, Thank you for this new day, its beauty and its light. Thank You for my chance to begin again. Free me from the limitations of yesterday. Today may I be reborn. May I become more fully a reflection of Your radiance. Give me strength and compassion and courage and wisdom. Show me the light in myself and others. May I recognize the good that is available everywhere. May I be, this day, an instrument of love and healing. Amen.(2)"

4. Call in all the Spiritual help available to you:

"I now call upon all my highest spiritual guidance and assistance available to me now and today to help me, guide me, elevate me, heal me, teach me, and protect me throughout my day. Thank you."
OR, you can also call in specific beings such as,

"I now call upon the Angels, Archangels, Dragons, Ascended Masters of the Highest Light, MY Spirit guides, MY Ancestor guides, to help me, guide me, elevate me, heal me, teach me, and protect me throughout my day today." (You can also use your own words)

5. Before leaving your home, apply energetic protection around yourself. Use one of the methods from Chapter 8 that resonates with you most.

6. Apply the energetic protection around your vehicle. If you take public transport, or get a lift with someone, apply it around those vehicles.

PM:
Evening routine before sleeping:

1. Clear your energy using one of the methods from Chapter 8.
2. Ask for help to clear the energy of your home using one of the methods from Chapter 8.
3. Thank your Spiritual team for all the ways that they helped you today. You can name them all or simply say *"Thank you to all of my highest Spiritual guidance and assistance that helped me today"*.
4. You may wish to add a prayer such as:

"Dear God, Thank You for this day. Thank You for my safety and the safety of my loved ones. As I enter sleep, may these hours give me peace. May they bring healing to my mind and body. While I sleep, dear Lord, please bless the world. Where there is pain, where there are people who have no place to sleep, who suffer and who die, may Your angels come unto them and minister to their hearts. Dear Lord, Please let the light stream in. Please use my hours of sleep. Please prepare me, during these hours of rest, for greater service to You. May the light that surrounds me, tomorrow shine through me. Soften my heart. Thank You, Lord. Amen.(3)"

5. Ask your Guardian Angel, or Archangel Michael of the Highest Light, to watch over and protect you while you sleep, both astrally and physically.

In addition to the above steps, try to also incorporate these Daily Actions into your schedule this week:

1. Move your body, preferably outside. Stretch, walk, hike, dance, take a class, whatever you like to do.
2. Ingest less chemicals through your food and beverage intake.
3. Always stay mindful throughout the day and conscious of your triggers. Jot them down in your journal so you can be aware of them.
4. Spend 10 minutes minimum in meditation or silence and stillness.

Optional:

1. Read a spiritual book that interests you.
2. If you'd like to start releasing your energy from unforgiveness, add this declaration to your morning routine: (you can also use your own words, the intention is what's important)

Forgiveness declaration:

"I (your full name), love myself and forgive myself on all levels, for everything that I did to myself in this or another lifetime.

I (your full name), love myself and forgive all the humans and beings, who have done something to me, in this or another lifetime.

I (your full name), love myself and and ask all the humans and beings for forgiveness, to whom I did something in this or another lifetime.

All chains and restrictions fall from me and I stand in my full power.

And so it is. And so it is. And so it is."
(Spend a moment after each sentence sensing the energy being released).

3. Purchase a deck of Oracle cards that resonate with you and pull a card each day for personal guidance.

4. Have another energy clearing and balancing session. Each session will go deeper, clearing away layers like onion skins.

Well done!

You've completed 21 days of new habits, new experiences, and brought new positive energies into your life. Please don't drop it all on Day 22. Instead, adjust it for your schedule, time and interests. Just go into each day remembering that you're a holistic Being and check in with your mental, emotional, physical and spiritual selves for any imbalance. Don't be afraid to call in your Spiritual team, remember they don't interfere so you have to ask them for help. And above all else, enjoy your life, appreciate the beauty that surrounds you, and prioritize yourself and your happiness.

Have faith in your wonderful shining self and personal power.

Prayers (1) (2) (3) are from this book; Illuminata, by Marianne Williamson

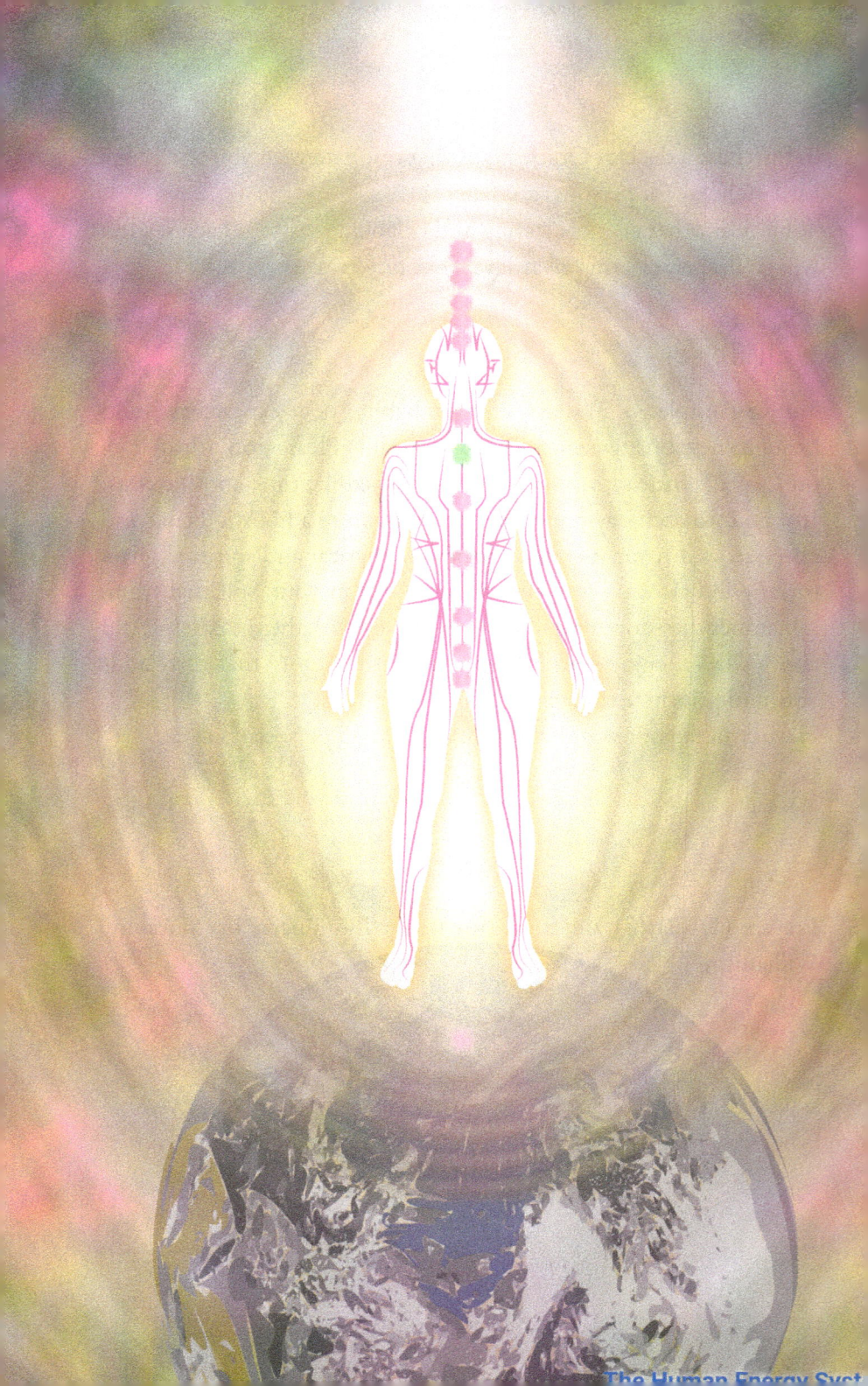

The Human Energy Syst

Brainwaves

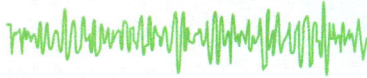

GAMMA
32-100Hz

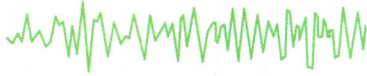

BETA
13-32Hz

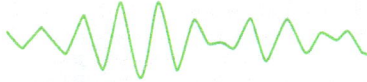

ALPHA
8-13Hz

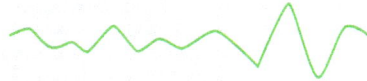

THETA
4-8Hz

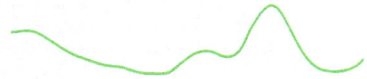

DELTA
0,5-4Hz

Side view of the main chakras

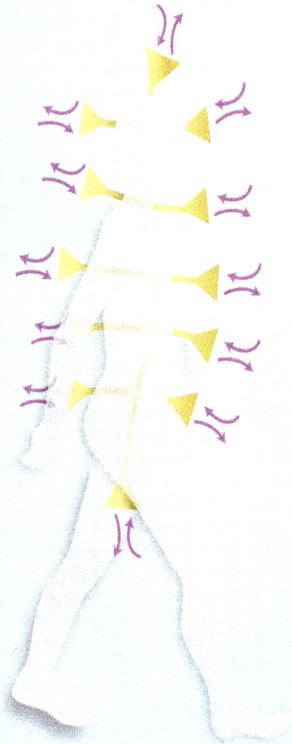

Water in the human body

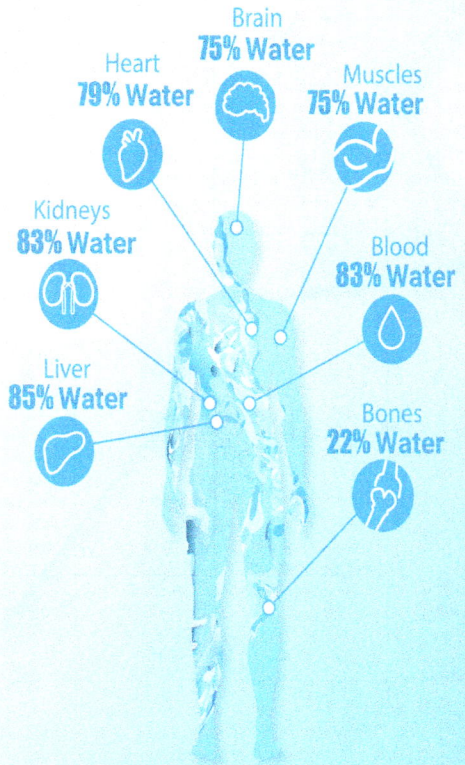

Brain
75% Water

Heart
79% Water

Muscles
75% Water

Kidneys
83% Water

Blood
83% Water

Liver
85% Water

Bones
22% Water

Chakra	Position	Associated Energy	Associated Organs & Gland	Archangel	Dragon	Common Crystal
Stellar Gateway	12" above the head	Bridge of light to higher dimensions and Source, Ascension pathway		Metatron	Suncaster	Calcite
Soul Star	7" above the head	Your Soul's knowledge from each lifetime		Mariel	Neptune	Selenite
Causal	slightly above the head	Communication with more Beings of light		Christiel	Christopher	Blue Kyanite
Crown	Top centre of head	A channel of connection to bring in higher spiritual guidance, Constantly channels Universal Life Energy into our system.	Brain, Nervous System, Pineal gland	Jophiel	Hesper	Clear Quartz
Third Eye	Centre of forehead	Intuition, Insight, Heightened sense of perception	Pituitary gland, eyes, ears, nose, nervous system	Raphael	Diogo	Amethyst
Throat	Centre of throat	Communication, Expression	Throat, Vocal Cords, Mouth, Lungs, Cervical Spine, Thyroid gland	Michael	Quicksilver	Lapis Lazuli
Dragon	Above the heart	Connection to Dragons and their energies				Jade
Heart	Heart	Love, Compassion, Understanding, Forgiveness	Heart, Blood, Lungs, Vagus nerve, circulatory system, Thoracic spine, Thymus gland	Chamuel	Analisa	Rose quartz
Solar Plexus	Centre of stomach area	Confidence, Self worth, Self empowerment, Willpower	Digestive system, Kidneys, Colon, Thoracic/Lumbar spine, Pancreas and Adrenal glands	Uriel	Drago	Tiger's Eye
Navel	below belly button	Oneness, connection to community		Gabriel	Saffron	Citrine
Sacral	Lower abdomen	Emotions, Sexuality, Intimacy, Creativity	Reproductive organs, intestines, Lumbar spine, Ovaries and Testes glands	Gabriel	Daphnae	Carnelian
Root	Tailbone	Basic needs; food, shelter, money, safety, security. Grounding	Bladder, Rectum, Genitals, Hops, Sacrum, Coccyx, Adrenal glands	Gabriel	Rufus	Smoky quartz
Earth Star	12" below your feet	Grounding and enabling you to fulfill your potential. Oneness with Mother Earth.		Sandalphon	Chameleo	Black Tourmaline

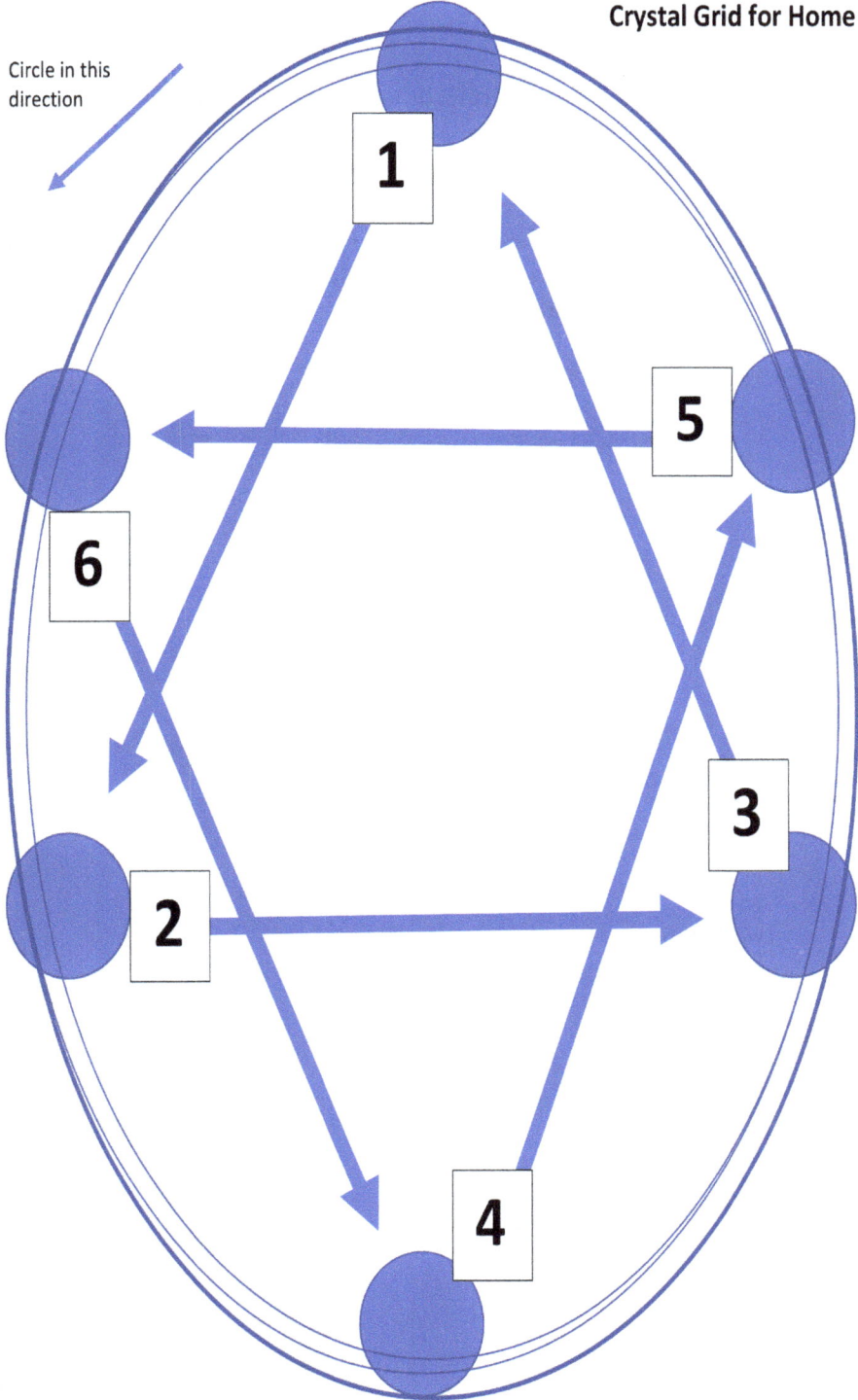

Crystal Grid for Home

Circle in this direction

Natasha Tomè is a natural empath and energy practitioner with multi-sensory abilities. A certified Reiki Master, Angelic Energy Master, Psychic Medium, Author, and Channeler of popular Guided Meditations available on YouTube, Spotify, Podbean, and Apple Podcasts. She communicates and works with the Spiritual Realm to bring in universal wisdom and energy for healing and guidance. She acts as a conduit to help people re-awaken and re-align to their true potential.

www.natashatome.com

Artwork Artist
https://auyantepuigrafico.blogspot.com/?m=1